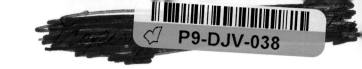

MEASURING
PATIENT SATISFACTION
FOR IMPROVED PATIENT SERVICES

AMERICAN COLLEGE OF HEALTHCARE EXECUTIVES MANAGEMENT SERIES

Anthony R. Kovner, Series Editor

Stephen Strasser
Rose Marie Davis

MEASURING
PATIENT SATISFACTION
FOR IMPROVED PATIENT SERVICES

MANAGEMENT SERIES
American College of Healthcare Executives

95 94 93 92 91   5 4 3 2 1

Library of Congress Cataloging-in-Publication Data

Strasser, Stephen.
  Measuring patient satisfaction for improved patient services / Stephen Strasser and Rose Marie Davis.
      p.   cm. — (Management series / American College of Healthcare Executives)
  Includes bibliographical references and index.
  ISBN 0-910701-78-4 (hardbound : alk. paper)
  1. Patient satisfaction.   2. Medical care surveys.   3. Medical care—Evaluation.   I. Davis, Rose Marie, date.   II. Title.   III. Series: Management series (Ann Arbor, Mich.)
  [DNLM: 1. Consumer Satisfaction.   2. Health Services—organization & administration—United States.   W 84 S89m]
RA399.A1S77   1991
DNLM/DLC for Library of Congress   91-20842 CIP

The paper used in this publication meets the minimum requirements of American National Standard for Information Sciences—Permanence of Paper for Printed Library Materials, ANSI Z39.48-1984.   ∞™

Health Administration Press
A division of the Foundation of the
  American College of Healthcare Executives
1021 East Huron Street
Ann Arbor, Michigan 48104-9990
(313) 764-1380

This book is dedicated to the following people, who care so much about our patient satisfaction project, the patients and staff it serves, and our lives:

Reed Fraley, director, the Ohio State University Hospitals; and assistant to the vice president of Health Sciences, the Ohio State University

Raymond Grady, president, the Evanston Hospital Corporation

Jan Berry Schroeder, director of Service Excellence, the Evanston Hospital Corporation

All of our Patient Satisfaction Measurement Team Members at the Ohio State University since 1988:

John Kennedy	Melissa Kramer
Chris Colian	Carol Holz
Karol Henseler	Sandra Stranne
Paula Reilman	Ryder Smith
David Wallace	Lynne Sexten
Susan Ashley	Catherine Vilareal
Bill Jennings	Linda Mattson
Sharm Devandra	Robert Dyckes
Greg Pauly	Candace Adams
Amy Moore	Laura Peters
Bob Schauer	Heidi Sebastian
Autumn McIntyre	Michael Deucher
Nancy Adams	

This book is also dedicated to my son, Wesley Ross Davis, who is one child born as a result of the "miracles of modern medicine," for his steadfast support of his mother. All that I am able to do and be is because of your love and grace.

CONTENTS

Acknowledgments ix

Introduction xi

**Part I   The Benefits and Costs of Patient Satisfaction
            Measurement**

1   Why Patient Satisfaction Matters   3
2   The Costs and Risks of Patient Satisfaction Measurement . . 27

Part II   What and Who Are We Measuring?

3   What Are We Really Measuring? 49
4   Learning about the Population We Wish to Survey 67

Part III   How to Measure Patient Satisfaction

5   The Layout and Design of the Survey 79
6   Writing Your Own Survey Items   91
7   Survey Distribution, Response Rates, and Sampling 113

Part IV   Analyzing Patient Satisfaction Data

8   Managing and Analyzing Quantitative Survey Data 129
9   Managing and Analyzing Qualitative Data 153

**Part V   Using Patient Satisfaction Data for Improved
            Patient Services**

10   Putting Patient Satisfaction Measurement Data to Work . . . 175

Epilogue 197

Appendix: Worksheet for Cost of Lost Revenues
            for Various Contingencies 199

Bibliography 203

Index 205

About the Authors 209

ACKNOWLEDGMENTS

Many people played a significant role in helping us write this book.

From the Patient Satisfaction Measurement Team at the Ohio State University we wish to thank Karol Henseler, Susan Ashley, and Sandra Stranne for their tireless editing, superb feedback, and commitment to making the book work. It is a privilege to work with such talented and positive people. Special thanks also to all the PSMS™ team members, whose excitement and energy over this project helped to motivate us.

Lee Bolzenius, the PSMS administrative coordinator, who did a fantastic job of keeping everything on the project running smoothly while we were completing the book during the summer of 1990, without question you are the best person we ever had the privilege to work with. Plaudits to Melissa Kramer, who joined our staff in December 1990 and who has contributed so much to the development and implementation of our system.

Many thanks to Tony Kovner, Ph.D., the Management Series editor at Health Administration Press, for his vision and for sharing our enthusiasm and excitement in the project. We greatly appreciate the support of all Health Administration Press staff for their thorough text editing and production expertise. Also, thanks to Larry Sachs, John Grima, Becky Rice, Jan Berry Schroeder, and an anonymous reviewer who offered a great deal of constructive feedback on an earlier draft of this book.

Jane Jordan Browne, you are indeed the best agent in the world! All of your efforts make our efforts at writing so much easier and more fun.

Our colleagues and staff at the Ohio State University's Division of Hospital and Health Services Administration deserve special mention. Their support, encouragement, and patience over the past ten years will never be forgotten. Specific thanks to Steve Loebs, chairman; R. J. Caswell; William O. Cleverley; Paul C. Nutt; Donald Newkirk; Sandra Tannenbaum; Sharon

Schweikart; and Bonnie Kantor. Our colleagues at the Ohio State University Hospitals were terrific as well. Special thanks to Cathy Bruno, Nancy Grover, David Irwin, Nancy Demaray, Lynn Greentree, and Mary Eleanor Jennings.

The College of Medicine at the Ohio State University has been in our corner from the start. Special thanks to Manuel Tzagournis, dean; Ron St. Pierre, associate dean; and Joan Patton, chief financial officer. Thank you for creating a work environment that so strongly encourages projects such as this.

Thanks to David Greenberger, our colleague at the Ohio State University College of Business, who kept the other projects going and whose research methods expertise and theoretical knowledge have contributed so much to the Patient Satisfaction Measurement Project. John Kennedy deserves special recognition for his development work with our qualitative coding system in 1989.

Last but not least, we wish to thank all the staff at the Ohio State University Hospitals and the Evanston Hospital Corporation. Their willingness to work so hard with us taught us more about patient satisfaction than they will ever realize.

This book was written with the goal of improving the quality of our patients' experience during their inpatient stays and outpatient visits. All of you mentioned above have contributed to this end. For this we are indeed grateful.

INTRODUCTION

In this book, we try to help health care managers improve the quality of the clinical and nonclinical services they deliver to their inpatients and outpatients. Our first message is simple: Measuring patient satisfaction can have a positive impact on your organization, your staff, and the patients it serves. In many ways, it represents your first step toward total quality management.

This book is not written for only patient and customer relations staff. Instead, this book is written for all health care managers—CEOs, assistant and associate administrators, medical directors, nursing vice presidents, clinical and nonclinical department heads, and academics; this book is as much about being an excellent manager as it is about patient satisfaction measurement. These are not mutually exclusive topics—in today's health care environment, great managers know how to learn about and manage one of their most important constituencies—their patients.

If you are like most managers we have met, then you are probably quite skeptical about whether patient satisfaction measurement systems can have such a dramatic impact. As one manager told us, "I never met a patient satisfaction measurement system that I liked!" Three years ago we probably would have agreed whole-heartedly with this manager. But opinions can change. Certainly ours did.

In the past few years we believe there have been some exciting developments in how patient satisfaction is measured and how the data collected can actually be used to benefit the health care organization, staff, and patients. Some of these developments focus on improved survey methodologies, while others focus on the specific integration of existing health care management information systems capabilities into the patient satisfaction measurement process. Ironically, many of these "new" developments are the piecing together of already available research methodologies and

xi

management information systems technologies. Moreover, they are eminently doable. Many of these technologies already exist, or they can be easily imported into today's health care organization. Our second message, then, is for skeptics only: Go ahead and remain skeptical, but you owe it to yourself, your commitment to being an effective manager, and your organization to take a new look at how patient satisfaction measurement has changed for what, we believe, is the better. In particular, please look at how the information it generates can make *you* a better health care manager.

If you are not a skeptic and you do believe in the efficacy of patient satisfaction measurement, then we hope we will offer you some new insights into this most critical managerial area.

What's in This Book?

This book is divided into five major sections. The first part is titled "The Benefits and Costs of Patient Satisfaction Measurement." In Chapter 1 we discuss the many ways health care organizations can benefit from conducting patient satisfaction measurement. Our approach is systems based; that is, the benefits extend well beyond learning only what patients think about their hospital stay or clinic visit—they can extend to the total organization. There are marketing, risk-management, organizational-development, fundraising, and even employee-recruitment benefits that must be understood and appreciated. Chapter 2 looks at the costs and risks of patient satisfaction measurement, and as importantly, how to manage, cope with, and minimize them.

The second part is called "What and Who Are We Measuring?" In Chapters 3 and 4, the theoretical and operational components of our model of patient satisfaction measurement are described. This part is important—it lays the foundation for sound patient satisfaction measurement. Moreover, some of the important methodological and technological approaches to state-of-the-art patient satisfaction measurement are described.

Part III is titled "How to Measure Patient Satisfaction." Chapter 5 focuses on organizing and designing your survey. Chapter 6 is a primer on how to write many different kinds of reliable, valid, and useful survey questions. Distributing your surveys, evaluating your response sample, and maximizing response rates are the central themes of Chapter 7.

The fourth part is called "Analyzing Patient Satisfaction Data." Do not panic. This is not about writing computer programs in COBOL or FORTRAN. Instead, it is a nuts-and-bolts approach to turning your data into useable, managerial-enhancing information. Chapter 8 deals with how to logically analyze numerical, or what we define as *quantitative*, patient satis-faction data. Chapter 9 addresses the management and analysis of the written comments patients provide in response to open-ended survey questions.

The fifth and final part is titled "Using Patient Satisfaction Data for Improved Patient Services." There is some purposeful redundancy in this part with Chapter 1, though new ideas are presented. In many ways this is the most important part of the book, since having unused patient satisfaction data reduce any system to meaningless dimensions. In Chapter 10, concrete managerial applications for patient satisfaction data are described in detail.

How to Use This Book

First, this book can be used as a resource book. It can offer, we hope, many useful ideas on how to conduct effective patient satisfaction measurement. Second, this book can serve as a launching pad for your own creative ideas and approaches to measuring patient satisfaction. Third, this book might affirm much of what you are already doing in the patient satisfaction area. Fourth, this book should be used as a tour guide to safely navigate you around and through the maelstroms of patient satisfaction measurement. Fifth, this book can help you justify (or not) in your own mind and the minds of others the potential utility of patient satisfaction measurement. Sixth, this book can help you and all your management staff to better communicate with two very important constituencies—your patients and your health care staff. Last though certainly not least, we hope that you use this book as a guide to being a better health care manager in general.

The Context, Ground Rules, and Limitations

This book is based largely on our experience with the Patient Satisfac-tion Measurement System Project (PSMS™), supported by the Ohio State University Hospitals; the Ohio State University's College of Medicine; the Evanston Hospital Corporation in Evanston, Illinois; the St. Vincent Medical Center in Toledo, Ohio; and the Upper Valley Medical Center, in Troy, Ohio. This project has been in effect for three years and is staffed by 12 graduate students, five Ohio State University faculty, and four full-time technical and administrative and support personnel.

The scope of this book goes well beyond our research project and our unique approach. A message we do not wish to send is that our approach is the only approach! It is our hope that you will use our model to better understand the totality of patient satisfaction measurement.

Examples used in this book are all masked to protect the anonymity and confidentiality of our survey respondents. At times the content of these examples are altered to attain this end. Nonetheless, the authenticity of these kinds of remarks is quite real. Any similarities to the actual comments of our survey respondents are coincidental only.

If you disagree with what we have to say, please let us know what you disagree with and why. This is one way we can further improve on the science and art of patient satisfaction. If a second edition of this book is published, then your comments may be included and duly noted.

This book contains innumerable suggestions and recommendations. It is critical that you review these in terms of their applicability and appropriateness to your own unique situation. We do not presume for a second that we have developed a flawless approach to patient satisfaction measurement that applies to all situations at all times. As we note throughout the book, there is still much to learn about patient satisfaction measurement, and we are among the first in line to learn.

There are some other limitations to this book that we would like to note. First, this book does not deal with the use of telephone surveying methodologies to evaluate patient satisfaction. This omission is not to suggest that these methodologies are inadequate. However, our experience is limited in this area. We believe that many of the topics we cover could apply to telephone surveying; however, we thought it best to stay away from a topic with which we have little practical experience.

Second, our treatment of this topic is probably biased in the direction of measuring inpatient satisfaction. Although the outpatient environment is discussed throughout, our focus is somewhat toward inpatient satisfaction measurement. This may not be a major problem since the principles underlying the measurement of inpatient satisfaction are often similar (though certainly not identical) to those underlying the measurement of outpatient satisfaction.

Third, much of our experience in patient satisfaction measurement is still quite new. Hence, all readers should be cautioned about the preliminary nature of many of our findings and recommendations. These caveats should be kept in mind when reading this book.

One final note: There is some (not a lot) purposeful redundancy in this book. There are a few reasons for this: Many of the topics we cover logically build on each other and transfer from one chapter to another. Also, some of the issues we address are fairly complex. Different examples of, and approaches to, essentially the same complex topic may help our readers better understand the ideas and content.

PART I

THE BENEFITS AND COSTS OF PATIENT SATISFACTION MEASUREMENT

1

Why Patient Satisfaction Matters

Patient satisfaction measurement matters for more reasons than health care managers may initially realize. A well-designed, implemented, and utilized patient satisfaction measurement system can help health care managers improve the quality of their clinical and administrative activities. Specifically, patient satisfaction measurement can be used to protect or increase patient revenues, conduct sound market research, improve risk management practices, build employee morale, document different levels of job performance, facilitate the performance appraisal process, improve the quality of care, and establish performance standards. If used to its fullest potential, patient satisfaction measurement can become a potent organizational development and strategic management tool for health care organizations in the 1990s and beyond.

We do not mean to sound like a television advertising hawker who in 20 staccato seconds tells America how "the amazing Wonder Gadget can carve, pare, shave, whittle, slice, dice, peel, cut, incise, cook, wash dishes, and do your taxes all for O-N-L-Y $19.95!" We intend to show you that the measurement of patient satisfaction offers tremendous potential benefits to health care managers for a relatively low cost.

In this first chapter, we will review many of the benefits of conducting patient satisfaction measurement. In the following chapters, we will look at the costs and risks associated with patient satisfaction measurement and how to manage and minimize these. Our premise for this chapter is not complex: Measuring patient satisfaction matters! Here's why.

Saving Lost Revenues

Consider the following case study:

Mary Smith came to Health Hospital for what was expected to be a routine delivery without any complications. The delivery was not routine, however, due to distress of the baby, and a cesarean was performed. After four days in the hospital, her physician, Dr. Jones, told her that she would be discharged within a couple of days. The baby was fine and she was recovering appropriately. Mary replied: "I can barely walk, and the incision hurts a lot when I try to move. How can I take care of my baby at home if I can't walk?" Her physician said in a derogatory voice, "You have a husband, don't you?" In reality, Mary was a single mother with no other support system available to her. After returning home, she received and completed her patient satisfaction survey from Health Hospital. Mary expressed her dissatisfaction with the physician's attitude and made direct comments to this effect.

Upon receiving her survey, Health Hospital's manager of Patient Relations called the distraught patient. Clearly, Mary needed a further forum and opportunity to vent her feelings and frustration. The patient representative apologized to Mary on behalf of the hospital and assured Mary that the hospital wanted to right this wrong. Even though there was little that could be done about Mary's situation, it was important that Mary shared her concern so that future patients would not be subjected to the same attitude and insensitivity. After asking Mary's permission, she was also assured that Patient Relations would speak directly with the physician so that he would be aware of how he had made one patient feel because of his lack of sensitivity.

After much listening and building a sincere trust with Mary, the conversation ended with Mary saying: "Thank you for calling me and listening—I really didn't know if anyone would pay attention to what I said or not. I never intended to return to Health Hospital for anything, but now that I have talked with you and know you are concerned about me, I'm willing to come back again."

Because of her initial dissatisfaction, Mary was going to initiate what Day and Landon classified in 1977 as a "personal boycott," that is, never return again—discontinue using the product or service (Singh 1988). What would have been the financial implications of this patient not returning to Health Hospital for the remainder of her life in terms of lost revenue for the hospital?

Unfortunately, there are not that many guidelines available in the literature to help us answer this question. A few models were brought to our attention, of which two (or rather one and a half) we were able to track down—phone calls to two sources yielded nothing, incidently! The first model is based on the work of Rosselli, Moss, and Luecke (1989). The second model, which this first model draws from, is based on the work of the Technical Assistance Review Programs (TARP 1983).

In light of this, we endeavored to develop our own model using the following sources of information:

1. Our own data from the Patient Satisfaction Measurement System (PSMS) (Strasser 1988)

2. Data from the above-mentioned article by Rosselli et al. (1989)

3. Data from the Healthcare Financial Management Association (HFMA 1989)

It is important to understand some of the limitations of this model before it is presented. First, the model is based on a set of assumptions that, of course, may not be valid or may be only partially valid. Second, our estimates of some of the model's parameters may also be less than precise. Furthermore, these estimates will be case specific; hence the average estimates employed may not capture a given hospital's actual cost of losing business from a dissatisfied patient.

To partially compensate for these deficiencies we have taken the following steps. First, we have attempted to be conservative in our estimates. Second, when we have reliable and valid data available, we employ them. Third, our model recognizes that there is a proportion of all dissatisfied patients who could never be satisfied, which we call the "uncontrollable dissatisfied." Fourth, our model accounts for the substantial difference between consumers' verbalized behavioral intentions (consumers stating that they will never go back again to a given hospital for medical care) and what they actually do. Finally, our model accounts for the large proportion of patients who, no matter how dissatisfied, may have no choice as to where they seek care.

General Assumptions

Assumption 1

At the very least, there is strong anecdotal evidence that dissatisfied patients talk (Rosselli et al. 1989). Specifically, they talk to other potential consumers about how unhappy they were with their health care experience. Obviously, bad-mouthing is negative advertising for the health care organization and tarnishes its community image and reputation. Moreover, it could influence a potential consumer's decision to use the services of the health care organization being criticized (Rosselli et al. 1989).

Assumption 2

Dissatisfied patients are more likely than not, to take their health care business elsewhere, assuming they have a choice. This, of course, means less revenue for the health care organization from this lost customer (it may mean fewer costs for the organization as well).

Assumption 3

Independent of choice, not all patients who holler "I will never return to this place again!" actually make good on their threat. There is ample research indicating that behavioral intentions are not always acted on. Offsetting this is that some who do not voice their complaints—the "silent dissatisfied"—will choose not to return.

Assumption 4

If the patient's dissatisfaction is resolved, chances improve that the patient will return to the same health care organization despite the original experience.

Assumption 5

Some patients are going to be dissatisfied no matter how hard the health care organization tries to prevent this (the "uncontrollable dissatisfied"). The "controllable dissatisfied" are patients whose judgments about their health care experience can be affected.

Assumption 6

The amount of revenue dissatisfied patients will cost a health care organization should they choose not to return will vary depending on the age of the dissatisfied patients, their health care status in the future, their type of insurance, and other sociomedical factors.

How Much Does It Cost to Lose a Dissatisfied Patient?

Given our strong cautionary comments about the validity of this model, let us consider one example of the revenues lost because dissatisfied patients choose to take their health care business elsewhere.

The following example assumes an urban hospital of about 450 beds with 14,500 discharges annually. It is further assumed that of those discharges, only 35 percent have a choice over where they seek inpatient care. Last, we are assuming that patients who choose not to return to the hospital that dissatisfied them would have experienced only one more readmission each to that same hospital in the future.

The model we designed is shown in Exhibit 1.1. "Soft" estimates are based on discussions with other health care professionals, logic, and intuition. "Hard" estimates are based on actual data collected in a systematic fashion. Obviously, we are more confident of the accuracy of the latter. Explanations for our estimates are given within the model itself. Please note that in the appendix different assumptions and estimates are used within the same model/framework.

Exhibit 1.1   A Model for Calculating How Many Dissatisfied Patients Will Not Return to the Same Health Care Organization for Care and the Associated Costs

Direct Dollar Losses from Dissatisfied Patients

Number of discharges per year	14,500	
Percent of discharges who have a choice over where they seek care	× 35.00%	("Soft" estimate based on discussions with health care professionals)
Total discharges who have a choice over where they may seek inpatient care	5,075	
Percent who say they will never return to the same hospital for care	× 2.48%	("Hard" estimate based on PSMS data, 1991)
Total number of patients saying they will not return	125.86	
Percent of patients who represent the "controllable dissatisfied"	× 90.00%	("Soft" estimate, which assumes that 10% of all patients can never be satisfied no matter what)
Total number of patients "controllable dissatisfied"	113.27	
Percent of patients making good on their threat of not returning	× 40.00%	("Soft" estimate based on the idea that behaviors occur far

Continued

Exhibit 1.1   Continued

		less than stated behavioral intentions. People often state they will engage in a given behavior, but then do not follow through.)
Total who actually do not return for their health care to the facility that dissatisfied them	45.31	
Lost revenue from inpatients who decide not to return, controlling for bad debt and contractual allowances	× $3,626	("Hard" estimate based on HFMA data, 1989)
Total lost revenues from nonreturning patients	$164,293	(Subtotal A)

Estimated Dollar Losses from Negative Word-of-Mouth Advertising

Total number of dissatisfied patients saying they will not return for inpatient care	125.86	
Number of people told by dissatisfied patients that the medical care was poor	× 6	("Soft" estimate based on Rosselli et al. (1989). Their suggested figure was 9 other people, which we reduced to be conservative.)
Total number of people who receive negative word-of-mouth advertising	755.16	
Percent who have a choice over where they receive care	× 35.00%	(See above)
Total number of people who receive negative word-of-mouth advertising and who do have a choice over where they seek care	264.31	
Percent of people who have a choice and will not choose the hospital based on the negative word-of-mouth advertising	× 12.50%	("Soft" estimate based on Rosselli et al. (1989), who suggest a more lenient figure of 25%.)

Continued

Exhibit 1.1 Continued

Total number of word-of-mouth group who will not use the hospital for medical care	33.04	
Lost revenue from inpatients who decide not to return, controlling for bad debt and contractual allowances	× $3,626	(See above)
Total lost revenue from patients who hear negative advertising and choose to take their health care business elsewhere	$119,797	(Subtotal B)

Grand Totals

Total lost revenue from dissatisfied patients who choose not to return to same institution (Subtotal A)	$164,293
Total lost revenue from potential patients who heard the negative word-of-mouth advertising and choose to go elsewhere for their medical care (Subtotal B)	+ $119,797
Grand total of lost revenue	$284,089

Note: The appendix applies the same model using different assumptions.

Critique of the Model

Why this example may be a conservative estimate

We believe our estimates are conservative in a variety of ways. First, our experience suggests that more (perhaps three times more) than 2.48 percent of all discharges feel as if they would never return to the same hospital again for treatment because of a dissatisfying experience. In fact, data on which this value is based are from a hospital that has superior high quality of care and patient satisfaction levels. What is more, patients' qualitative (written) evaluations of their stays often suggest a deeper level of dissatisfaction than is expressed in the quantitative (numerical check-the-box) section of the survey evaluation form. Moreover, patients sometimes tell us they are far more satisfied than they really are. Criticizing one's health care provider can be, in the eyes of the patient, risky business. In effect, some patients tell us nothing, but are seething inside and are going to be undercounted in this model. If the percent of patients who say they will never return is raised to 5 percent (from 2.48 percent), then the total lost revenue figure increases to roughly $572,000 (see the appendix at the end of the book).

Second, we believe our estimate of the number of "uncontrollable dissatisfied" is somewhat high. It is unlikely that 10 percent of the dissatisfied patients cannot be reasoned with.

Third, we have made no provision for malpractice suits, which could be more likely among dissatisfied patients. If only one patient among the 2.48 percent who say, "I will never go back *there* again," sues and wins, then the financial implications could be substantive.

Fourth, the model assumes that dissatisfied patients will experience only one more hospitalization for the remainder of their lives worth $3,626 to the hospital. Rosselli et al. (1989, p. 22) assume five admissions "in a patient's remaining lifetime." Moser (1991) estimates approximately two admissions, with a length of stay of five days each from middle age on.

Fifth is the issue of choice. In the above example, we assume that 35 percent of the inpatient population have a choice about where they seek inpatient care. As noted earlier, estimating this value is extremely difficult because consumers' ability to choose will be a function of their insurer, sociodemographic factors, physician, and medical condition. However, if that figure were to be raised to 45 percent, then the total amount of lost revenue is about $409,000. If the percent of patients who say they will never return is also raised to 5 percent (from 2.48 percent), then the total lost revenue increases to about $825,000.

Finally, certain costs that could have dollar implications were not included in the model. For instance, dissatisfied patients can take up enormous amounts of staff time. What's more, they can create serious psychological stress and morale problems for employees. The dollar value of both these factors could be substantial.

Why these estimates may be deceivingly high

There are factors acting in the opposite direction that would decrease the cost of losing dissatisfied patients to another hospital. For instance, suppose this hypothetical 400-bed urban hospital had the finest customer relations program in the country. Even under this circumstance, some controllable dissatisfied patients will still choose to take their health care business elsewhere. Hence, in the above example, it would be impossible to recoup all of the lost dollars.

Second, the total value of lost dollars is deceiving because these are not net dollars. The hospital may be losing $284,089 dollars in revenue for a given year, but then again it is not incurring any variable costs on these lost patients. Hence, the marginal benefit of keeping a patient's business needs to be weighed against the marginal cost of providing the care.

Third, to be technically accurate, we should also take into account the timing of the lost dollars. Patients who choose not to be readmitted a year after their dissatisfying inpatient stay will not have associated with them the same present value cost as patients who choose not to be readmitted 12 years later.

Fourth, our estimate for the percentage of patients who will actually follow through on their statement, "I will never return," may be somewhat high at 40 percent. If that figure is lowered to 30 percent and all other estimates stay the same, then total lost revenue drops to $243,016. However, if any of the other estimates were to be simultaneously increased, then the total revenue loss figure would rise substantially.

Fifth, we recognize that the model does not account for duplicate patient visits, which will inflate the value we use to estimate the number of patients who will choose not to return.

What Can We Conclude?

In light of all the caveats and cautionary comments, the following conclusions might be tentatively drawn:

1. It will cost the health care organization if it loses a dissatisfied patient to another institution. The exact amount is unclear. What is clear is that if enough of these patients go elsewhere, it can hurt your business. Viewed from a slightly different perspective, one might argue that, at the very least, dissatisfied patients are not likely to help the health care organization in any way.

2. When intangible costs are brought into the equation, such as a better organizational image due to fewer patients publicly bad-mouthing the organization, less internal stress among staff due to dissatisfied patients, and fewer "Mobile Videocam Newswatch Channel 78" stories about angry health care consumers, the cost savings could grow even more.

3. Increased market share has become a major objective for many health care organizations. Logically, one could argue that dissatisfied patients are not going to contribute to attaining this goal.

4. Many health care managers, whether they realize it or not, seem to believe that satisfied patients will result in dollar gains. How else can we explain the time, energy, and money that is poured into

patient satisfaction enhancement programs like valet parking, VCRs in patient rooms, and customer relations training for all staff?

5. If dissatisfied patients can hurt your business, then it becomes crit-
    ical to have some formal method of identifying who these people
    are, measuring what harm was done to them (from *their* perspec-
    tive), measuring what the depth and intensity of their dissatisfaction
    is, identifying where this occurred in the health care setting, and
    identifying how the problem can be remedied. In short, patient satis-
    faction measurement becomes as necessary as financial accounting,
    human resource management, and medical staff relations!

With a large dose of prudence and caution guiding our assessment, we believe that there are meaningful dollar implications in patient satisfaction measurement.

Benefits for Your Health Care
Organization's Marketing Program

Health care marketing managers would be wise to view patient satisfaction measurement as a potential treasure chest of market research and marketing opportunities. We will look at some of the market research implications first.

Market Research

The process of patient satisfaction measurement provides market researchers with an excellent opportunity to answer relevant research questions. This can be done by looking at the patient satisfaction survey in a multidimensional way.

On one level, a patient satisfaction survey is designed to measure how patients feel about their hospital experience(s). At another level, survey questions can be designed for market research purposes and then added on to the patient satisfaction instrument.

There is an operational elegance to this idea that should be noted. Many patient satisfaction measurement systems sample their population of discharged patients on a quarterly basis. Hence, for a 300-bed hospital, approximately 3,000 discharges (12,000 annual discharges/4 quarters) are surveyed annually. This is an excellent market research sample that should not be underutilized. In fact, the survey can be altered each quarter so that comparative field studies on marketing issues can be conducted.

Here's how this idea might be implemented by health care man-agers. Suppose health care managers are interested in obtaining a current assessment of their consumers' needs and expectations. Open-ended questions, like the following, could be easily placed at the end of a patient satisfaction survey:

- Please list two ways in which you would like to see the medical services at Health Hospital improved.
- Please list one major aspect of the medical care you received at Health Hospital that makes you want to return should you need medical care in the future.

Closed ended market research questions could be employed as well. Consider the following examples.

- Would you be more likely to use our outpatient clinic if we offered valet parking at a cost of $3.00 per visit?

  ____ Yes ____ Maybe ____ No
- Below is a list of new patient services we are thinking of offering at Health Hospital. Please check off those you feel would make it more likely for you to use Health Hospital.

  ____ Free shuttle service for outpatient appointments from your home to the hospital

  ____ Bedside video players and free movies for entertainment in the hospital

  ____ Hospice care for cancer patients

  ____ Open visitation hours for family members

  ____ Banking services for hospitalized patients

  ____ Child care for small children during adult outpatient appointments

Note that in the last example, rank-order methodologies could be applied as well.

Suppose the market researcher is trying to evaluate the "climate" or "image" of a hospital from the patient's perspective. Semantic differential scales (Moser and Kalton 1972) could be included in the patient satisfaction survey as follows:

- We want you to express your general impressions of Health Hospital. Circle the number below that best expresses how you feel. Health Hospital is:

Friendly	←	1	2	3	4	5	6	7	→	Unfriendly
Cozy	←	1	2	3	4	5	6	7	→	Intimidating
Big	←	1	2	3	4	5	6	7	→	Small
Hard to get around in	←	1	2	3	4	5	6	7	→	Easy to get around in
Indifferent	←	1	2	3	4	5	6	7	→	Caring

Using patient satisfaction surveys as a tool for marketing research does have its limitations. One methodological concern is "external validity," that is, the extent to which research results are generalizable (Campbell and Stanley 1963). Specifically, who is to say that discharged patients reflect the true composition of the larger population you are trying to measure? This is a valid question. The results from these add-on market research survey items can be generalized at best only to discharged patients. However, this is a population in which most health care managers are interested. Today, patient satisfaction survey measurement can be designed to measure and analyze, in a valid way, demographic information of respondents (and nonrespondents), which then allows researchers to assess, in part, the representativeness of their sample. Moreover, other market research that is conducted by the health care organization can be used to cross-validate the results of these add-on items.

A second potential limitation is that the add-on items could confound the responses discharged patients give to the portion of the survey that deals specifically with their health care experience. Care in the design of a market research survey section obviously needs to be taken.

We are not suggesting that patient satisfaction measurement can replace all market research methodologies. Rather, we believe that patient satisfaction measurement can be a logical and relatively inexpensive way to begin to answer a variety of market research questions.

Using Survey Data for General Marketing Purposes

Patient satisfaction measurement generates data that offer marketing personnel extremely useful information. For example, patient testimonials on the excellence of their care can be abstracted from these surveys and, with the respondents' written permission, used on promotional materials. Consider the following example:

> I was a high-risk pregnancy and this was our first baby. We were absolutely petrified! We had just walked on eggshells for the last nine months to make this happen. The nurses in Labor and Delivery were so sensitive to what Andy and I had gone through to even get to the

point of having this baby that they really made it the most wonderful experience of our lives. Jason Randolph is now four weeks old and is healthy and delightful. Thank you, Health Hospital!

This is a marketing dream: Imagine the positive word-of-mouth influence in the community and the return potential of this couple for their next baby and other services to Health Hospital!

Patient satisfaction performance scores can be used for the same purpose. For example, suppose a group of ambulatory care settings called "Health-in-a-Moment's Time" ran a patient satisfaction survey and learned that 95.7 percent of its survey respondents agreed that they would recommend Health-in-a-Moment's Time to family and friends. These data can then be reported in subsequent advertising campaigns.

The marketing department of a hospital can get even more sophisticated with the data it reports for external and internal promotional purposes. Consider the following example: A medium-sized hospital implemented a thorough patient satisfaction survey after much work and thought. After 16 months of collecting data, an upward trend in perceptions of patient satisfaction over time was identified (Figure 1.1). Consider the potential impact

Figure 1.1   A Graph Constructed for Internal Purposes

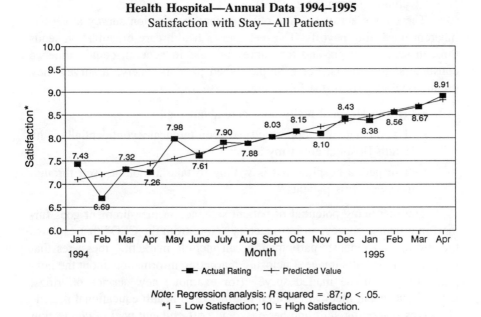

Health Hospital—Annual Data 1994–1995
Satisfaction with Stay—All Patients

Note: Regression analysis: R squared = .87; p < .05.
*1 = Low Satisfaction; 10 = High Satisfaction.

Figure 1.2   A Graph Constructed for Advertising Purposes

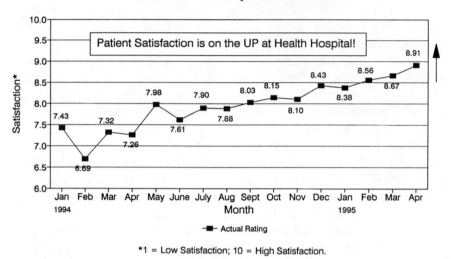

Health Hospital—Annual Data 1994–1995
Satisfaction with Stay—All Patients

of this kind of graph constructed for advertising purposes, that is, without all the technical jargon (Figure 1.2).

The simple act of sending out a patient satisfaction survey alone has inherent marketing payoffs: The messages a health care organization sends through survey design, and the survey process in general, could influence consumers' judgments. For example, when patients receive a survey they might conclude any of the following:

- "Health Hospital really does care about me."
- "I appreciate the opportunity to communicate confidentially with Health Hospital about my hospital stay."
- "I respect a hospital that is willing to take a look at itself through the eyes of its patients."

The marketing potential of patient satisfaction measurement goes further. In a mailed survey, an introductory "Note from the CEO" that explains the survey and requests participation can include marketing messages that bolster the hospital's image. Enclosing marketing information about the hospital along with the mailed survey (for example, new service offerings, news about recent medical research findings, and health educational materials) gives marketing staff another easy and cost-efficient way of connecting with the consumer. Take care to ensure that these materials do not interact with the judgments discharged patients are asked to make about their recent hospitalization. Otherwise, the patient satisfaction data could become contaminated.

Benefits for Your Risk Management Program

Patient satisfaction measurement systems can help improve the quality of your hospital's risk management program. Here are some suggestions on how this can be accomplished.

Triaging (Prioritized Screening) of Incoming Surveys

When patient satisfaction surveys are returned, a designated hospital employee can be trained to review or "triage" all of the written comments (and scan the numerical scores) on the surveys within 48 hours of receiving them. If these comments (or scores) are like any of the following, a hospital representative can flag and respond to them in a timely fashion (the patient's name and medical record number can be encoded on the returned survey or voluntarily recorded by the respondent), allowing for direct follow-up:

- "My wife's an attorney. You'll be hearing from us!"
- "I'm suing!"
- "I received awful care at your hospital, and I have been trying to reach my doctor to complain about it. Not only will she not return my phone calls but your hospital's patient relations office won't return them either. I wouldn't return to your hospital if my life depended on it!!!"

Triage protocols can be created along a variety of dimensions. One model might employ numerical "screens." Here, patients with satisfaction ratings below certain values would be classified as "high priority." More complex models might be created as well. Cunningham (1987) of KCA Research indicates that patients sue because of

- Lack of communication
- Lack of continuity of care
- Delay in action
- Accessibility/responsiveness
- Expectations unrealized
- Professionalism lacking

These factors could easily be adopted as additional criteria on which triage classification decisions are made. The keys to the triage system protocol just described are that the surveys are (1) reviewed and then flagged within 48 hours of receipt and (2) responded to by a patient relations representative immediately. If hospital management can quickly respond to these high-priority concerns, then we believe it will be less likely that these patients will speak ill of, or bring suit against, the health care organization. Moreover, many of these patients may have very valid complaints, which may indicate a larger problem in the organization's administration of care. Identifying these problem areas permits management to take necessary action to solve these problems before other risk management problems emerge within the health care organization.

But what about the person who does not fit the "squeaky wheel" profile—the person who is dissatisfied but is not ranting and raving about revenge and lawsuits? A well-developed patient satisfaction measurement system can compile the names and telephone numbers of patients who have indicated low levels of satisfaction. This group can then be contacted by hospital personnel to see what the hospital can do to rectify the situation. For example, at the Ohio State University Hospitals and the Evanston Hospital Corporation, we have trained managers to telephone patients whose surveys indicate a specified level of dissatisfaction. Managers ask these discharged patients what the hospital can do to improve their situation, and then the managers contact the hospital's patient relations office if any follow-up is needed. Early results suggest this program is promising. It is described in detail in Chapter 10.

Improving the Productivity of Employees

Accountability

Companies such as Northland Dodge, Wendy's, Kinko's Copy Centers, General Motors, and the Hyatt Regency Hotel frequently survey how satisfied their customers are with their services. Although there is nothing enlightening or innovative in the idea of a customer satisfaction survey itself, surveying consumers sends company employees and managers a very important message: You are being evaluated. Instantly, health care staff who have contact with consumers are placed on notice that the consumer is looking directly at their performance to see if they are doing their job effectively. In addition, management is looking over their employees' shoulders via the returned surveys for exactly the same reason. This instills in employees a feeling of performance accountability—employees are now more easily held accountable for their job performance. By the same token, managers are held accountable for the employees working with them.

From a management perspective, this is crucial. Patient satisfaction measurement requires health care professionals to make a cognitive connection between their attitudes and behaviors and how they will be perceived by patients (the consequences). Health care professionals who have had a long and grueling day may now be more likely to think to themselves: "I'd better watch out how I behave during this last hour of work with my patients. I feel stressed, and this could come across to my patients. If I'm curt with someone, I could get written up!"

Twenty years ago, some health care professionals might have indulged themselves in inappropriate customer relations behaviors without much risk. Today, patients are taking names, literally. They are writing down the names of employees and managers who are behaving improperly and informing patient representatives, their physicians, and management.

With increased accountability should come increased job performance. Nurses may now behave more patiently to those incessant questions that family members ask because they know that patients will be asked to respond to the survey question: "Was your nurse responsive to your family members' questions?" Dietary employees may be more concerned about presenting the food in a timely and appealing manner, knowing that patients will be asked to evaluate the quality of food services. Some physicians may now take a few extra minutes to really listen to their patients because they know they will be evaluated on this.

Some may believe that current survey methodology is not precise enough to pinpoint individual providers who deliver poor services. They are wrong. By utilizing a sophisticated patient satisfaction survey system, providers will no longer be allowed to hide behind the protective shield of anonymity. The methodology currently exists to break down survey results into areas such as nursing discharge unit, nursing shift, medical service, admitting and attending physician, and so on. From our experience, many patients are writing on their surveys in-depth comments, both positive and negative, about their health care experiences. Moreover, they are doing this willingly.

In sum, patient satisfaction measurement creates a strong incentive for employees and managers to improve upon their performance and to maintain high levels of performance. It is not just a system of negative incentives—the health care staff is trying to avoid being written up; rather, positive incentives can be offered that will encourage high levels in employee performance.

We do not want health care managers after reading this section to think, "Now I can catch all my people doing the wrong things I know they're doing and document it!" Such Machiavellian thinking is antithetical to how appropriate patient satisfaction measurement systems should be used. These systems are used for far more than only accountability and performance evaluation purposes. They should also be used as a tool for administering performance-contingent rewards and identifying ways in which patient services and medical care can be improved.

Goal Setting

Patient satisfaction measurement can be used in goal-setting programs, which, in turn, may also result in higher job performance (for an in-depth discussion, see Chapter 10). For example, work groups can set patient satisfaction performance targets for themselves and then evaluate, on a monthly or quarterly basis, how they have fared. In this way, patient satisfaction measurement becomes an organizational development tool. What is more, patient satisfaction performance standards should be tied into the health care organization's overall quality assurance system. For instance, nursing unit 3 East might set the following target:

> On the survey question "The nurses responded promptly to my calls," 3 East will *never* have a quarterly score below 3.50 and will identify 3.75 or higher as our target goal for 1993 (where 1 = Strongly Disagree and 5 = Strongly Agree).

Nursing administration can then monitor this on an ongoing basis. When positive or negative deviations from the goal occur, the administration can work collaboratively with 3 East to see why things have taken a turn for the better or worse on that unit.

Improving Organizational Climate and Employee Morale

As mentioned previously, not all the news from a patient satisfaction measurement system is bad. From our experience, most of it is very good, if not excellent. The large amount of positive feedback generated can be used in a variety of helpful ways.

Recognition

First, it can be used to recognize high-performing employees. Lack of recognition is a major complaint among health care employees. How often have you heard members of your staff bemoan, "They (management/physicians/regulators) only tell me what I'm doing wrong around here, never what I do right." Patient satisfaction measurement can aid in solving this problem because patients on their satisfaction surveys frequently name individual health care professionals that they feel did a terrific job. These names can be compiled in a data base and then posted throughout the organization, published in a newsletter, or both. The desirable behavior the patient is commenting on can, and should, be linked to the health care professional's name:

> Judy Marcuse, the LPN on 4 North, was the most caring nurse I have ever met. I was feeling enormous discomfort at night after my surgery, and she stayed with me and held my hand until I was able to fall asleep again.

Feedback on Excellent Job Performance

Improvement in patient satisfaction may also be used to help build a positive work climate for the health care organization as a whole or within its departmental subgroups. Suppose dietary services were to receive the information shown in Figure 1.3 from a longitudinally trended patient satisfaction survey. The impact of this feedback on most any work group would be positive. Contrary to popular opinion, working people do want to know how they are doing on the job (often, they just do not like how they are told). Positive feedback of this kind will go a long way toward making the work group feel good about itself and the job they are doing.

Improving Quality of Care

Reliably and validly measuring quality of care has been the focus of much academic, practitioner, and regulatory attention over the past 20 years. Today, most believe that "quality of care" is a multidimensional concept. For instance, it is not uncommon to see the quality formula defined in terms of multiple indicators, such as nosocomial infection rates, unplanned readmissions within 30 days of discharge, mortality rates, and negative deviations from standard protocols of treatment.

In recent years, patient satisfaction has been added to this list of quality indicators. The Ohio State University Hospitals and the Evanston Hospital Corporation represent two examples of this. Of the twenty-one quality assurance (QA) indicators the former hospital monitors monthly, three of these are patient satisfaction measures: satisfaction with overall care, satisfaction with nursing care, and satisfaction with physician's care. If a hospital's patient satisfaction measurement system is not formally a part of the QA system, then patient satisfaction is still reviewed as though it were a QA indicator. We believe there are at least two factors that have contributed to elevating the status of patient satisfaction measurement to that of a QA measure.

Figure 1.3 Example of a Graph that Can Be Used to Provide Feedback
on Job Performance

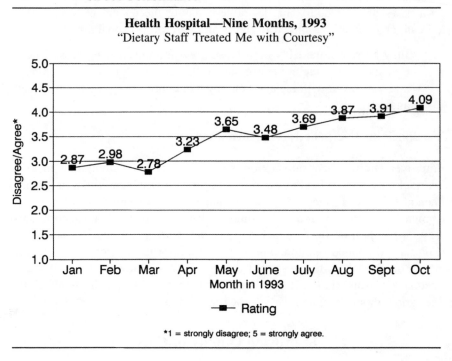

Health Hospital—Nine Months, 1993
"Dietary Staff Treated Me with Courtesy"

*1 = strongly disagree; 5 = strongly agree.

First, the definition of quality has been expanded to include many
of the service delivery aspects of care—responsiveness, courtesy, dignity,
maintenance of confidentiality, sensitivity, waiting time, and so forth.

Second, the patient is no longer considered a naive and uninformed
observer of the quality of health care rendered. Health care managers are
now listening to patients' perceptions of how competent staff appear, whether
staff behave professionally, and, more to the issue, how treatment was delivered. Today, for instance, if only one patient indicates that he or she believes
that a provider is impaired by alcohol, alarms go off—very loud alarms—
and many of us have seen this happen. Measuring patient satisfaction, then,
has added a whole new perspective to the quality-of-care formula.

Patient satisfaction measurement also can contribute to increased quality of care because the patient can often identify problem areas of which
management is not aware. Management may know, for instance, that their
admissions process is slow. However, they may not realize the depth and
intensity of the problem or how detrimental this can be to the patient's

well-being until they read a comment from a patient satisfaction survey like this:

> They told me to report at 9:00 A.M. I didn't get into my room until late that afternoon—over eight hours later! That's why I was crying. That's also why my husband was enraged.

When this kind of comment becomes a common occurrence, management knows they have a major problem in admissions that must be resolved. One could argue that just one comment like this is a problem.

The quality of care can also be improved because innovative ideas for improvement are often offered by patients in their satisfaction surveys. For example, prior to the opening of a new cancer hospital, a terminal cancer patient sent in her patient satisfaction survey and described how difficult it had been for her family members to adhere to visitation policy hours. The family lived about 45 miles from the hospital, and between travel time and visiting hours, it had been very difficult to coordinate seeing the patient as much as they had wanted, since she was going to die within the next few months. This patient suggested that there should be open visitation hours for all cancer patients, not only when there is a terminal condition, because of the general fear associated with having "cancer." As a result of reading this and considering with sensitivity the needs of this patient, the new cancer hospital's visitation policy is open hours, 24 hours a day.

An obstetrics patient returned her survey with comments concerning how difficult it had been for her when she went to her routine checkup in her eighth month and her doctor told her that they needed to deliver the baby immediately because the baby was in distress. She had come to this visit with her two other children, ages two and four. Her husband was out of town on a business trip, and she had no relatives or any close friends to call to take the other two children immediately. The staff watched the children until the husband arrived at the hospital after he was notified. The patient suggested that an emergency child care program might be useful for similar situations in the future so that valuable staff time would not be used to babysit and so that small children would be in an appropriate environment. This suggestion was taken to heart, and a program was implemented in conjunction with a nearby day care center for this type of care. These ideas offer a wealth of information that could have positive impact on quality and overall improvement.

We believe that patient satisfaction measurement might improve quality in at least one other way. Asking patients to evaluate their health care experience formally legitimizes them as active members of the health care delivery team, making them more involved and interested in all aspects of their care. It may encourage them to report their condition more readily, as well as those aspects of their medical treatment that could affect their well-being. For example, a patient might ask a nurse, "Should the saline solution bag connected to my IV be empty for over two hours? I mean, is that okay?" Increased involvement can pay dividends in terms of the quality of care and services delivered.

Benefits for Your Development and Fund-Raising Efforts

Within the last decade a viable alternative revenue source for hospitals has been private contributions. Many not-for-profit hospitals have consciously and aggressively established separate development (fund-raising) functions within their organizations with an eye on capital, contingency, and operational support dollars.

It is noteworthy that based on national figures analyzing who gives, how they give, why they give, and how much they give, personal, individual contributions account for a little over 82 percent of all of the philanthropic dollars (White 1986). Of all charitable contributions, 14 percent are made to health-related causes.

Obviously, a target audience for any development officer in health care should be the individual patients of that hospital. How does the development officer decide which patients to approach? All hospitals know who their VIPs are and who the potential largest gift givers are, but what about the patients? It is here that the patient satisfaction survey system can be employed. Patients who have indicated high levels of satisfaction with the health care organization can be downloaded from the data set and then contacted for gift-giving. If the patient satisfaction measurement system is sophisticated, then patient names can be further sorted along a set of criteria, like age and zip code, that could have a bearing on their ability to give.

Using patient satisfaction measurement for fund-raising is not without certain risks. In addition, there are ethical considerations to weigh as well. These are discussed in depth in Chapter 10 and must be considered if your organization is planning to institute such a program.

Conclusion

The system of health care in this country is no longer a one-way, top-down relationship, commencing with the provider and ending with the consumer. It is a reciprocal relationship, which the health care organization must nurture in order to maintain and improve quality and to remain competitive. This is certainly consistent with current thinking on total quality management.

Health care organizations that do not believe that what their patients have to say matters are living in the dark ages of health care management. They are clinging to the age-old adage "The doctor (provider) knows best"—true only from an unenlightened health care organization's narrow perspective!

2

THE COSTS AND RISKS OF PATIENT SATISFACTION MEASUREMENT

The costs and risks of patient satisfaction measurement are not trivial. They must be fully understood by health care managers in order to either avoid them, or to manage them effectively. If accomplished, the potential benefits of a patient satisfaction measurement system grow exponentially.

In this chapter we will identify some of the major costs and risks of patient satisfaction measurement. In addition, we will suggest ways these can be reduced or effectively managed.

The Dollar Costs

The first question most health care managers ask when deciding whether to implement a patient satisfaction measurement system is, "How much will it cost us?" The answer to this question will be frustrating: "It depends!" It depends on the depth and breadth of the system that you put into place. The following cost estimates are based on having an outside consulting firm run most aspects of your patient satisfaction measurement system.

This is not meant to suggest that health care organizations cannot conduct their own patient satisfaction surveying. They can, and some do it very well. However, our experience is with the contract research we conduct for other health care organizations, and we feel safer reporting from our own experience. Moreover, it may make more sense for many health care organizations to contract with outside firms and academic institutions for this work because they may not have the staff, technology, experience, and computer hardware and software to do it well.

One final note about the cost estimates given below. We offer these estimates with *great trepidation*. They are just that—estimates. They are based on our experience, which may or may not be similar to others'. In addition, we are presenting only a broad-based accounting of the cost of patient satisfaction measurement. Getting into the detail of every line item would, we believe, be distracting and unproductive. However, if you contract with a firm for patient satisfaction measurement services, make sure you do ask for detailed, line-item pricing.

The Deluxe Model

For a deluxe system, which includes the following components, the annual price tag could run as high as $6.00 per discharge, whether all discharges are surveyed or not. For $6.00 per discharge, the health care manager could expect the following services from a consultant:

1. A tailor-made survey, unique to the needs of the organization. The survey would be about 70–100 items long, attractively laid out, and printed to maximize user-friendliness and response rate.

2. Surveys mailed to every discharged patient, and return postage on the surveys paid by the consultant as well.

3. Medical record information encoded on the survey (for example, patient's DRG, age, sex, medical service, nursing discharge unit). This involves accessing information from the patient's medical record, preferably within a week of discharge, and then encoding it onto the survey via a mailing label or direct printing. This task is not as simple as it may sound!

4. Detailed feedback reports six times a year with graphics and a variety of statistical breakdowns (for example, patient satisfaction by patient age, sex, and nursing discharge unit). Brief data summaries during off months could be provided.

5. Triage of incoming surveys to identify potentially serious risk management incidents.

6. A patient satisfaction survey of nonrespondents conducted annually. *Nonrespondents* are defined as patients who fail to respond to the first round of distributed surveys. This type of survey helps establish the generalizability, or lack thereof, of the initial group of respondents.

7. Analysis of the written patient comments (qualitative analysis) and their systematic coding and classification.

8. In-depth training of hospital staff in how to interpret and *use* the patient satisfaction survey data.

9. Longitudinal trending of quantitative and qualitative data with norms provided, and advanced statistical analysis, such as factor analysis of scales, regression analysis, and causal model building.

10. Patient mix–adjusted satisfaction scores (statistically adjusting satisfaction scores to account for a hospital or clinic that treats, say, a younger or older patient population). This results in far more accurate intergroup/interhospital comparisons.

11. Biannual feedback sessions to senior management on the results of the surveys.

12. Close integration of the survey process with the health care organization's patient relations staff.

Hence, a 300-bed hospital that discharges 12,000 patients per year would pay approximately $72,000 per year for a deluxe system. A 600-bed hospital doing 24,000 discharges per year could expect to pay about 1.8 times as much, or $129,600 (some savings may accrue due to volume). Although these costs may sound high, consider them as a percentage of the hospital's total budget. If a 300-bed hospital has an $80-million budget, then $84,000 represents one-tenth of one percent of the total. One wonders if Sears, Bell Telephone, and Hyatt spend this little on finding out what their customers think and feel.

The Midline Model

For a middle-of-the-road system—the midline model—a hospital could expect to pay about $3.50 per discharged patient. The following services would be included:

1. A boilerplate survey, with minimal tailoring to the health care organization's unique needs.

2. Surveys mailed to every discharged patient for only four- to six-week sampling periods annually; that is, every third or fourth month, the total population of discharged patients are surveyed for four to six consecutive weeks.

3. Quarterly feedback reports with detailed graphics and a variety of statistical breakdowns based on the patient's age, sex, acuity, location of stay or visit within the hospital or outpatient clinic, and so on. Encoded survey methodologies would be employed.

4. Triaging of incoming surveys to identify potential risk management incidents.

5. General analysis (for example, typing only) of the discharged patients' written comments (qualitative analysis) and no systematic coding and classification of these comments.

6. Limited training of hospital staff in how to use the patient satisfaction results.

7. Longitudinal trending for quantitative data but not for the qualitative data. Norms provided.

8. Patient mix–adjusted satisfaction scores for better intergroup comparisons, as previously discussed.

9. Annual feedback on survey results to senior management.

Here, a 300-bed hospital with 12,000 discharges a year will pay about $42,000 annually for this service. Similarly, a 600-bed hospital will pay about 1.8 times more, or $75,600. These costs would represent about one-twentieth of one percent of the hospital's overall budget.

The Economy Model

What about a "beater" or a low-budget model? For this program, expect to pay about $2.00 per discharge; however, expect to get very little in return. You may, in fact, get so little that you might not want to even waste your time and money on this. There are many reasons why.

First, it becomes virtually impossible, at this price, to analyze qualitative data—the patients' written comments. Without this analysis, the efficacy of the system is undermined since the qualitative data often hold the more useful and insightful information about the patient's stay. Second, at this price, the "unit-of-analysis problem" rears its ugly head. To be useful, patient satisfaction measurement data must be broken down beyond simply overall hospital trends. Overall hospital trends are useful, but limited. To find out specifically what is going on in a health care organization, the unit of analysis must be smaller and more specific. Today's health care manager can have patient satisfaction results broken down by DRG, medical service, nursing discharge unit, primary or attending physician, length of stay, and nursing shift (see Chapters 8 and 9). Qualitative data analysis and specified unit of analysis feedback are not cheap; however, the potential benefits to health care establishments are immense.

We wish to reiterate that these cost estimates are, of course, presented with great trepidation. They are very rough, and they may not account for many other factors that will affect—positively or negatively—the total cost estimate. In addition, the cost estimates provided should be lower in the second year of a new system. Some of these charges are incurred only during the first year—survey design, computer programming, developing reporting systems, and staff training.

Ways to Reduce Dollar Costs

Are there ways to reduce these costs? The answer is yes. However, be very careful of reducing the quality of your product and overburdening your staff because you wish to save money.

The first trick is to do much of the work yourself. Substantial cost savings can be accrued by implementing the following steps. Please note again that these are estimates only:

1. Design your own survey. Some health care organizations have staff who are sufficiently trained in survey research to develop their own instrument. Simply reviewing the literature on patient satisfaction measurement will get an inside staff person off to a good start (Meterko, Nelson, and Rubin 1990). However, a word of caution is called for. Designing surveys properly is much more difficult than one might originally think. When we say you need "trained staff" in survey research methodologies, we mean, *trained staff*. Potential savings could amount to about $3,000 to $5,000 in the first year.

2. Conduct all the mailing yourself rather than pay for someone else's overhead. Hospital volunteers, for instance, can stuff envelopes and handle the mailing process. Potential savings could amount to $2,000 annually.

3. Conduct the triaging function yourself. Training a staff person to read and triage all the incoming surveys is relatively easy to do. In at least one way, this is the preferred method: it expedites the triage process since the surveys do not have to go to a consulting firm first. Potential savings could amount to $2,000 to $3,000.

4. Ask for only raw data feedback from the consulting firm you are working with, and conduct the report writing and graphical analysis yourself. The report-generating task can be time intensive and costly, especially if sophisticated statistical and written analysis and interpretation are included. Having your own staff do this will save about $700 per report generated. In this way, you will save approximately $8,400 with a 12-month reporting system, and $2,800 with a quarterly system.

5. Conduct your own in-house training on how to use the patient satisfaction survey feedback. Potential cost savings could amount to
   $3,000 to $6,000.

6. Conduct your own feedback to senior management. Potential cost
   savings could amount to $3,000 per feedback session.

7. Conduct your own longitudinal trending. Potential cost savings
   could amount to $1,000.

If you add all of this up, the cost savings are substantial, ranging from
about $17,000 to $26,000 annually, depending, of course, on how often you
survey and the size of your facility. In effect, the outside consulting firm
is doing only data organization and data entry—entering the raw surveys
into a data base management system. Of course, many hospitals could do
this function, as well. However, in the interests of quality control, this is
probably not advisable unless you are sufficiently well staffed to manage
and conduct this function.

What you may lose as a result of these cost-cutting steps are norms—
the ability to compare your hospital to other similar institutions. However,
this cost is, in part, offset once you begin to generate longitudinal data.
Although norms are good, the best comparison you have is your own hospital
or outpatient clinic (and its subsystems/units) compared to itself over time.

A second caveat is that someone still has to do the work. While you
may not be paying a consultant $5,000 to develop your survey, an in-house
staff member will now have to allocate a great deal of time to doing this
task.

The question of who should quarterback the survey will come down
to principally three factors:

1. Do you have the in-house staff with the technical know-how to
   design and implement a sound system?

2. If so, are you willing to pay the opportunity costs of having in-
   house staff work on patient satisfaction measurement rather than
   something else? Our experience is that some managers tend to un-
   derestimate the conceptual and operational complexity of patient
   satisfaction measurement. If you are going to rely on your in-
   house staff to design, implement, and maintain your system, then
   be certain that you fully understand the difficulty of successfully
   conducting patient satisfaction measurement. The fact that so many
   health care organizations today do retain outside firms to operate
   their systems suggests that many managers have learned just how
   time intensive and difficult measuring patient satisfaction can be.

3. If an outside group does the work, it will be easier for the health care organization to credibly say to its public that these are "objective" and "independently" gathered measures of service and clinical quality.

Heightened Expectations

Any time a health care manager surveys people about their feelings about anything—their boss, job, pay, physician, nurses, parking accessibility, and benefit packages—an implicit and potentially dangerous message gets sent: If you take the time to tell us in your survey how you honestly feel, we will do something about the issues and concerns you raise.

The surveyor may not intentionally send this message, but, unless properly managed, the message gets sent through the survey process itself. The result is that health care consumers may have heightened expectations that the hospital will take action on the problems they have cited. Consumers who respond to patient satisfaction surveys may think that the insensitive nurse they were subjected to will finally be sent to a seminar entitled "Ten Ways to Be Nice," hospital bills will suddenly become easier to interpret and the food service will expand its menu to include lobster. "After all," thinks the consumer completing the survey, "if they didn't plan to do something about their problems, why would they bother to ask for my opinion in the first place?"

The problem of heightened expectations becomes critical when the same patients (or their family members or friends) are readmitted and the problems still exist. The hospital or outpatient clinic has implicitly promised to do something about the problems, yet they remain. Broken promises yield low trust. Broken promises yield consumers who feel betrayed. Low trust and feelings of betrayal may cause consumers to go elsewhere for their medical care.

Ways to Manage Heightened Expectations

First, we must accept the fact that the problem of heightened expectations can never be completely resolved, only partly managed. Here are some suggestions on how to do this.

Lower consumer expectations

Mailed surveys often have introductory language in a cover letter or on the survey itself that explains the survey process. We recommend including a disclaimer such as the following:

Health Hospital takes your comments very seriously. All of your returned surveys will be carefully reviewed, and your written comments will be closely read. Although we cannot promise to resolve every problem you raise, we at Health Hospital will do the best we can to resolve as many problems as possible.

The phrase "cannot promise to resolve" may serve to keep consumer expectations somewhat in check.

Managers must take action!

Before management commits to conducting patient satisfaction measurement, they must make one crucial commitment: Management will take action on at least some of the survey results that suggest corrective action is needed. If management is unwilling to do this, then they are wasting their own—and their patients'—time, a lot of money, and enormous amounts of energy. Although they may believe that they are enhancing the institution's image, since they are communicating one-on-one with their patients, the lack of corrective action behind these words is likely to undermine the credibility of the organization and its management in the eyes of consumers. Board members at cocktail parties will hear from patients and their family members and friends such comments as, "You know, my mother was just in your hospital again, and the food service is still lousy. Didn't anybody read her patient satisfaction survey? What are you people doing there?"

Not only must management take action, but they must *link* the action they take to the patient satisfaction survey feedback they have received. We cannot emphasize enough the importance of this point. Suppose Health Hospital decides to offer videocassette rentals because patient surveys indicate that patients, family members, and friends thought that this might be an excellent addition to traditional in-room television. This decision can be presented to the public—via signs, articles in the hospital's magazine or newsletter, or marketing materials—in one of two ways:

- *Message A.* "Health Hospital now offers videocassette rentals. Dial 2–VIDEO and you can have your favorite movies or children's cartoons in your room in just minutes."

- *Message B.* "Based on feedback we received from our patient satisfaction surveys, we have started offering videocassette rentals. Dial 2–VIDEO and you can have your favorite movies or children's cartoons in your room in just minutes."

The difference between the two messages is due to *cognitive linkage*. Message A simply indicates that a new service is available. Message B explains that this new service is available and, as importantly, that it is the result of the hospital taking action in response to patient satisfaction survey results. The power of making this type of linkage salient is potentially substantial. Here's why.

First, the credibility of the survey process is enhanced because management can demonstrate that they are actually using survey results to improve the quality of services and care at Health Hospital. Second, management can now demonstrate that, when good ideas are suggested, they will take action to implement them; a precedent has been set. Third, management is demonstrating that they not only take action, but that they also perform the necessary antecedent step—they really listen. For example, skeptical survey respondents may sometimes write or think, "I am responding to this survey and telling you honestly what I think about my recent hospital stay; however, I know no one reads these things." Management, patient relations, and marketing can now respond to this person by saying pleasantly, "I can understand why you feel this way; however, Health Hospital does care. How can I help you?"

Resistance to Patient Satisfaction Measurement: Morale and Organizational Climate

There is at least one immutable law in the workplace: Evaluation of job performance breeds anxiety. Patient satisfaction measurement can all too easily undermine good organizational climate, and the reason is simple: No matter how you package it, present it, and wrap it, patient satisfaction measurement is a form of evaluation. Moreover, for many health care staff, it is the worst kind of evaluation—evaluation by the "uninformed" patient.

This is not to say that all health care staff gag at the thought of patient satisfaction measurement. Nothing could be further from the truth. Many welcome the process and view it as a way to professionally grow and develop, and to improve patient care. However, evaluation may seem threatening to health care staff. Staff members are likely to assume the worst when discussions commence about implementing a new patient satisfaction measurement system. Fear of losing their job and lowered economic viability, looking bad in the eyes of their boss, and losing personal control over their work are likely to head the list of concerns among health staff. Let's explore the source of some of these concerns in more depth and from a few different perspectives.

The Physician's Perspective

Some physicians will feel threatened by patient satisfaction measurement. There are a variety of reasons for this—some good, and some not so good.

First, physicians may be frightened of receiving a "bum rap"—being held accountable for an outcome over which they have no control. This reaction is justified in many cases. For instance, a patient may complain on a survey that she was in terrible pain, and that she blames her doctor for this. However, with some medical conditions, this cannot be avoided without jeopardizing the quality of care rendered.

Second, some physicians may be fearful that the truth about their doctor-patient relations (DPR) skills, or lack thereof, will become documented. No physician would welcome the knowledge that they treat their patients with less dignity and respect than any other physician in the hospital. In outpatient settings, some physicians are abusive of patient waiting times—they may double-schedule their appointments. A well-designed survey will pick up this information quickly because the physician's name may be printed by patients on their surveys. Remember, patients in the 1990s are taking names.

Third, and at a more psychological level, some physicians will be threatened by the loss of control that patient satisfaction measurement brings. Now, more so than ever before, physicians are being held accountable to a much larger constituency—their patients. Moreover, patient satisfaction measurement potentially means "meddling" by management in their already harried and stressful life. Now the medical director, an old medical staff ally, will be coaching colleagues who score low on the DPR portion of the survey on how to be more responsive and more courteous to their patients.

Fourth, as is true with so many other professional groups, physicians may resent being evaluated by lay consumers. Many physicians may think, "If my patients knew what it was like to see 35 patients a day on four hours of sleep, then they would be a little more understanding about my seeming so rushed and impatient." While lay evaluation of professional services is nothing new to the 1990s, many physicians and other health care professionals still cling to the feeling that only they and their peers can make valid, reliable, and fair judgments of their performance.

Finally, we have met with physicians who feel that patient satisfaction measurement could represent a substantive legal threat should a malpractice claim, for example, be filed. Perhaps these physicians fear that the survey will be treated in court as an accurate testimony about their behaviors and attitudes.

The bottom line can be resistance to patient satisfaction measurement. Like so much evaluation, physicians may view survey data as information that can only hurt, not help.

The Manager's Perspective

Management's anxiety over patient satisfaction measurement stems from some of the same factors already cited, in addition to some others.

Management's anxiety, and subsequent resistance, is, in part, related to the inherent limitations that constrain their scope of ameliorative action. They may truly wish to take corrective action on negative patient satisfaction survey feedback, but often they are unable to do so. Lack of resources, such as time, dollars, and staffing, will always be an obstacle to implementing many of the solutions they believe will work. The net result is that management can look bad in the eyes of all of their constituencies: medical staff, nursing, the board, the press, the community, and their peers.

This issue takes on even greater significance when management tries to explain why they cannot act. An unsympathetic board or medical staff may scream, "Excuses, excuses. All we hear are your excuses!" As one very excellent and proven manager said to us when she was considering implementation of our patient satisfaction measurement system, "You're going to make my life miserable. Your surveys will identify a lot of problems that I'm not going to be able to fix. Yet, I'll still be held accountable for them." Perhaps, there is logic in the age-old adage "Ignorance is bliss."

This problem roots itself more deeply when health care managers need to intervene in problem clinical areas (for example, a problem nursing unit) because often they have only indirect control over those personnel. If the clinical head is not supportive, then the manager's ability to take positive action is dramatically reduced. The catch–22, however, is that again management may be held accountable.

Second, like physicians, management staff may learn they are not doing as good a job as they thought or hoped in certain operational areas, again perhaps reflecting badly on them and leading to heightened feelings of job insecurity.

Third, patient satisfaction measurement forces the manager to work with bad news. For instance, names of providers and staff who are not behaving appropriately with patients will appear on surveys. Although the health care manager realizes that it is helpful to be able to identify problem providers and staff, it is not fun having to address the problem. In fact, one of the hardest tasks for a manager is to confront employees with poor job performance.

Fourth, management may fear the negative climate that patient satisfaction surveys can create. In one organization, the patient satisfaction surveys became known as the "complaint form." This is not the kind of working environment and culture that health care managers wish to create.

The Nurse's Perspective

Nursing will experience many of the same concerns noted above. The concern over lay evaluation of nursing job performance will be foremost in their minds. So too will be nursing's concern about not being able to respond to the problems that emerge from the survey. Here the biggest issue may be centered around staffing. We can hear nursing managers sincerely saying after receiving survey feedback results, "I know we should be spending more time speaking with the patient's family about their loved one's condition. However, we're so short-staffed, we simply don't have the time for that. While we're trying to provide the best care we can for our patients, their families are rating us as rude and indifferent, and I can understand why."

The Perspective of Dietary and Environment

Dietary's and Housekeeping's resistance to patient satisfaction measurement may be grounded in their knowledge of the predisposed negative bias most people have about hospital food and sharing a room with another patient.

It is no secret that throughout the history of hospital care in the United States, dietary and room environment have been the traditional scapegoats for patient and family member frustrations. Think for a moment about all the bad and often unfair jokes people make about hospital food and environment:

- "When are they letting you out of jail?"
- "My pain would be all gone except for the food."
- "The only roommate I can live with is my wife!"
- "Mmm, looks delicious—for my dog."

Anxiety and concern over the patient satisfaction measurement process from staff in these two sectors of the organization should come as no surprise.

Managing Resistance and Fear

Use patient satisfaction survey data positively with your health care staff

Many of these anxieties will blossom if health care professionals feel that patient satisfaction measurement will be used to "thin out the ranks," "weed out the bad ones," and "get rid of the fat." Specifically, if health care staff feel that patient evaluations are being used primarily in a negative and punitive manner, then there is little doubt that anxiety, resistance, and fear will run deep. To quote Dr. William F. Jessee of the Joint Commission on Accreditation of Healthcare Organizations in a speech at a conference on "The Service Quality Connection" in May 1990:

> The challenge of quality improvement is to try to measure how well we're doing in meeting our customers' requirements, not as a means of identifying who's screwing up and punishing them, but rather as a tool for us to figure out where improvements can be made. This is a different philosophy than we've been operating under in the recent past.

Here are some steps that management can take to ensure that patient satisfaction measurement is used positively.

First, management will need to take the philosophical and public position that the purpose of patient satisfaction measurement is not to harm the hospital's or clinic's staff. In addition, the message must be sent that the system will be used for many of the positive reasons cited in Chapter 1— setting performance targets, finding ways to improve performance, positive feedback, and sharing good news.

What management says and does must be consistent. If management chooses to put on notice department heads whose initial patient satisfaction evaluation returns are poor, then they are undermining the purpose and efficacy of the system. If, however, management sits down with their department heads and tries to collaboratively figure out how to solve problems defined through patient surveys, then their actions are reinforcing their words.

Like all evaluation, properly managing the feedback process is as crucial as the design of the evaluation itself. Jaundiced organizational members may think, "Sure, this is what they're saying, but if my name keeps coming up in complaints, then I'm history here." Management's response is relatively easy. If employees, after repeated efforts at rehabilitation, are unable to "clean up their act," then they should be fired. The employee pulled the trigger, not the patient satisfaction measurement system.

Special attention should be given to identifying the appropriate person who should give feedback—positive or negative. If a physician's name keeps coming up as "Dr. No the Nasty," then management needs to sit down with the medical director or chief of staff and discuss who should give the feedback to this physician and how. When nursing is involved, obviously nursing should take the lead on feedback. For clinical departments, the department head with clinical skills and expertise would be the logical choice if clinical issues are raised.

Working smarter, not harder

Receptivity to patient satisfaction measurement will increase if it can help hospital staff work smarter, and not necessarily harder. Suppose nursing unit 3E on weekend shifts at Health Hospital is consistently coming up with very low patient satisfaction scores. In particular, this unit rates the poorest on the survey question pertaining to responsiveness to patient calls. There could be a variety of factors responsible for this outcome: higher acuity, poor staffing, lazy nurses, overreliance on less well-trained nurses, and so on. After some investigation, nursing management may conclude that the nurses are not lazy and that the true cause of the problem lies in inadequate staffing patterns. Hence, with enlightened management, the results of patient satisfaction surveys may, in fact, result in smarter management decisions and better allocation of resources. The results are not always going to be management pointing an accusatory and adversarial digit at slothful and negligent employees.

System design

One of the best ways to allay evaluation anxiety is to allow those affected by the evaluation to be involved in the design of the system. This applies to patient satisfaction measurement directly. Hospital and clinic management would be wise to involve physicians, nurses, ancillary staff, business office staff, and others in the design of their patient satisfaction measurement system. Although pluralistic system design can be frustrating and painfully time-consuming, it most often proves to be worth it in the long run.

If health care staff are not consulted, then their needs for professional autonomy and self-determination are violated. The result may well be an excellent patient satisfaction measurement system that never gets off the ground because the process of developing it was mismanaged. Again, the *process* of evaluation is as important as its *design*.

Information sharing

Another good way to allay evaluation anxiety is to make sure that those affected by the evaluation are allowed to review the actual survey results. For instance, the vice president of nursing would get to see all of the relevant nursing information on a quarterly basis. However, this alone is not enough. Senior management, in turn, must then share unit-specific, shift-specific, and service-specific data with their lower-level managers and staff. In this way, the feedback of patient satisfaction survey data is no different than the way the results of employee attitude surveys are handled.

Protecting egos and staff confidentiality

Patient satisfaction data can become more useful when it is compared to some other group, standard, or norm. Although deliciously tempting perhaps, be very careful about this. First, never show one department/unit head another department/unit head's patient satisfaction performance scores. This is akin to publicly sharing performance evaluation information. Moreover, it is an ethical violation—you are breaching both department heads' confidentiality. Naturally, the department head with the lower patient satisfaction measurement scores will be upset at his or her relatively poorer performance, and publicizing the information makes the situation even worse. This, in turn, could lead to resistance to the entire patient satisfaction measurement process. What's more, such comparisons may be grossly unfair. For instance, one could argue that comparing patient satisfaction ratings of hospital pharmacists to those of hospital lab staff is like comparing apples and oranges. After all, pharmacists usually relieve pain, while laboratory personnel often inflict it—no matter how hard they try to do otherwise.

Be a good researcher

Good researchers are painfully aware of the limitations of their work. When researchers are up-front about this and, at the same time, follow justifiable research practices, the academic and practitioner communities' willingness to listen to what they have to say will increase. Managers using patient satisfaction feedback should treat it exactly like research data—handle with care. Like good researchers, health care managers must have an intimate understanding of the limitations of their patient satisfaction measurement system. If health care staff believe that management views their patient satisfaction feedback as blinding and unequivocal truth, then they will be gun-shy of the evaluation process. On the other hand, if employees know that management is aware of flaws and pitfalls in patient satisfaction measurement, then their resistance should, in part, wane. Here are some of the limitations that should be kept in mind by management when interpreting patient satisfaction data.

First, patient satisfaction data represent only one perspective of job performance—the patient's perspective. Obviously, this is not a foolproof measure of how well hospital and clinic staff perform. Recent research in the area of cognitive psychology has repeatedly proven that observers (here the patient) can be biased in their perception. Cognitive psychology aside, management must also consider the medical and psychological status of many of the patients and how this can add even more error into the process. After patients take a pain medication such as Demerol, they are often unable to recognize where they are, let alone be able to make accurate judgments about the medical care they are receiving. Moreover, as health care professionals frequently argue, the patient may not be a perfect judge of clinical treatment quality. Clearly, judgments by the health care professional's manager and peers also need to be factored into the overall performance equation.

Second, some patients do not always understand context. Nurses may be doing an outstanding job responding to call buttons in light of the heavy acuity and staffing shortages on their floor. However, these patients may not soften their criticism or enhance their praise in light of this. After all, some patients may have no idea of the context.

Third, the data from patient satisfaction surveys may not be representative of the total population of patients served. Management must keep this in mind before making generalizations and drawing conclusions about what patient satisfaction results mean. If sample sizes are small, management should have less confidence in the data. The message here is, interpret data feedback with caution.

The lesson is clear: Patient satisfaction is a critical part of the total quality-of-care and job performance puzzles; however, it is only one of many parts. If used alone or overweighted in the evaluation of performance, then health care professionals will chafe at it.

A devil you know is better than one you don't

Like most people, managers hate to get blindsided. How often have you heard managers say, "If I had only seen it coming," or "Why didn't you tell me that the patient who waited eight hours in admissions was a board member's son *before* the board meeting last night?"

One of the best ways to justify patient satisfaction measurement is to persuade management that ignorance is not bliss when it comes to the evaluation of patient satisfaction. Although managers may have trouble solving the problems patients cite, it is in their best interest to know about them as they happen and before they become even more widespread. At the very least, an effort toward damage control of a very difficult problem is always a better performance strategy than looking into your board president's or CEO's eyes and saying, "I just wasn't aware this was a problem. Honest!" This kind of ignorance in the 1990s does not spell *bliss*, but rather *job termination*!

The Ethical and Value Risks of Patient Satisfaction

All management information system data can be abused, and patient satisfaction data are no different. Previous sections of this chapter discuss how patient satisfaction data should not be used as a sledgehammer poised for descent over low-performing employees' heads. But how about patients and their families? Are there ethical risks health care managers need to be aware of?

In this section we will focus only on the ethical issues and risks of patient satisfaction. The legal implications of patient satisfaction measurement will be discussed in the following section.

Ethically, who owns the data?

The answer is that the patient owns the data. When patients return their survey they are giving the hospital or outpatient clinic the *privilege* of reading what they had to write about their care. This privilege should never be abused.

Should a doctor be shown an individual survey from an identifiable patient who indicated he or she was treated horrendously?

The answer is NO! The patient's right to anonymity and confidentiality must be protected. Many patients would feel betrayed, even horrified, if they found out that their close family doctor (and friend) learned what they had written about them on their survey in confidence. Not only is this unethical, it's lousy research. How can we expect patients to honestly express how they feel if they have even the slightest doubt that their confidentiality and anonymity will be violated?

Does this mean doctors will never be told about their very unhappy patients?

Of course they can, and should, be told about negative comments written about them. However, physicians should never be told which patient in particular made such comments. Moreover, no information should be divulged from the survey that in any way could identify the source of these negative comments. However, if the patient specifically says, "Tell my doctors and nurses exactly what I wrote—word for word," then you should call the patient and verify if this is indeed the patient's wish. If the patient confirms, then go ahead and share the information with the providers identified.

Does the same hold if the comments are positive or good?

Yes, we can share the good news, but not the source of it or any information from the survey that could identify the source.

How careful do we need to be about protecting the patient's confidentiality and anonymity?

Extremely careful. The information contained in the patient satisfaction survey should be treated no differently than the information contained in the patient's medical record. All people involved with the survey process, from secretaries opening the surveys sent by return mail, to data entry operators, to patient representatives, must be trained in the ethics of patient satisfaction measurement. The survey and the data must also be located securely. Only those trained in the ethics of patient satisfaction measurement should have access to individual surveys.

Should some patients not be sent a survey?

Good question! First, think very clearly about whom you wish to receive the survey. For example, a patient may die in the hospital, but, somehow, the patient's name shows up on the mailing distribution list. When the survey is mailed to this person's home, you may receive a justifiably angry phone call from the family member or friend who opened the envelope in which the survey was mailed. In short, do not send surveys addressed to patients who died in the hospital! Obviously, some patients may die after they leave the hospital, and the hospital may have no knowledge of this. Although this could create problems, we have not faced any based on our own experience.

Second, be very careful with obstetrics patients. You can run into at least two kinds of disasters here. Since both the mother and newborn receive a medical record number, it is possible to send two surveys to the same household, one to the mother and one to the baby. Although the mother would obviously discard the baby's survey, you would look somewhat foolish and unprofessional by not controlling for this in your mailing distribution system. Also, be very careful not to send a survey to a mother whose baby lived for, say, a few hours or days after birth, only to die shortly thereafter in the hospital. These and other sampling issues are discussed in more depth in Chapter 7.

What if the data are not reviewed and used by the hospital?

Collecting patient satisfaction surveys and allowing them to collect dust is unethical, as well as a waste of scarce resources. As noted earlier, the act of surveying implies, at the very least, that the surveys will be read and the feedback will be seriously considered. How would you feel if you spent the time to tell someone how you truly felt and he or she was listening to a

Four Tops cassette on a Walkman while you were speaking? This is how patients will feel if they discover that their surveys are not even being read.

Legal Risks

In today's health care environment, practically everything poses a legal risk. Patient satisfaction measurement is not immune. Patients who feel their confidence was breached during the patient satisfaction evaluation process could sue. Also, after receiving a survey, the hospital could promise to follow up with a patient over a clinical matter. If no follow-up occurs and the patient suffers, then a suit could be brought. Such possibilities are endless. Despite this, you may solve more legal problems than you create by conducting patient satisfaction measurement (see Chapter 1, where risk management is discussed in depth).

One way you can minimize your legal exposure is to have the health care organization's attornies work with you in the design and implementation of your system. They can sensitize you and your staff to potentially litigious situations. Also, have your attorney work with your system on an ongoing basis. This is important from a risk management perspective.

Another possible way to minimize risk in using the information is to follow the rule, When in doubt, ask patients for permission to use their survey.

Although there are clear-cut legal risks to patient satisfaction measurement (as is true with most anything else in this world today), it is our belief, not empirical judgment, that patient satisfaction measurement is a relatively low-risk endeavor as long as the ethics of the process and sound research methodologies are employed.

Bad Data and Wrong Data

Botching the data collection, data input, and data analysis processes inherent to patient satisfaction measurement is an important risk to be considered and avoided at all costs. Most health care managers probably have no idea just how easily an unreliable, invalid survey can be designed, or how easily the computer programs used to analyze these data can be flawed. We shudder at the amount of misinformation that is probably created in this way. Worse yet, think of all the wrong decisions that could be made because the information base used is wrong. Although this topic is discussed in much more depth in Chapter 8, the following ideas will begin to give you some ideas on how to protect against these problems:

1. Get professional help in the design of your survey. Everyone believes they can design a good survey when, in fact, few people can.

2. Pretest your system thoroughly on a small sample of discharged patients.

3. Spend time and money on ensuring the quality of your data. Besides good survey design, it is important to develop quality assurance protocols for the whole data entry, data throughput, data analysis, and data feedback processes. It is worth repeating that miscodings in computer programs or poorly designed coding schemes alone can reduce an otherwise good system to meaningless gobbledygook. Again, make sure your system has stringent internal quality assurance standards.

4. Operate off of the philosophical premise that the data are wrong until proven otherwise. The contradictory philosophy of "innocent until proven guilty" is one of the fastest paths to inaccurate survey research.

Conclusion

After reading this chapter, health care managers may be shaking their heads thinking, "This is just not worth the cost or the risk." We believe that nothing could be further from the truth and that the cost-benefit ratio for patient satisfaction measurement will typically fall in favor of the benefits. Again, what is one repeat customer worth to you? How much do angry customers cost you in dollars, staff time and morale, and goodwill? What is one prevented malpractice lawsuit worth to your hospital? Please review Chapter 1 for the answer to these questions.

The reason we spend so much time on costs and risks to effective patient satisfaction measurement is simply to improve the chances of these benefits accruing for you. Remember, a devil you know is better than one you don't!

Last, though certainly not least, while many of the risks and costs of patient satisfaction measurement have been highlighted in this chapter, our list is certainly not exhaustive. Our best advice to health care managers involved in patient satisfaction measurement is to always think through the consequences of any patient satisfaction decision they may make or of any action they may take.

PART II

WHAT AND WHO ARE WE MEASURING?

3

WHAT ARE WE REALLY MEASURING?

In this chapter, we will first explore the concept of patient satisfaction. Specifically, we will try to answer this question: When we are talking about measuring patient satisfaction, what are we truly trying to measure?

Although you may be tempted to skip this chapter because you think it will be boring, anyone involved in the health care field should find it interesting. It is important because developing an excellent patient satisfaction measurement system requires a sound understanding of the concepts being measured.

In the last section of this chapter, we will briefly review ways in which health care managers can go about measuring patient satisfaction.

What Does Patient Satisfaction Mean?

Let us begin by having you, the reader, participate in a very brief exercise. Please set aside the book and take a few minutes to write out your definition of patient satisfaction.

How did you do? If you gave this exercise some thought, then it probably did not go as easily as you initially might have expected. Perhaps you thought you had a workable definition, and then you realized that it was not comprehensive enough; it did not capture the full meaning of the patient satisfaction concept. Some of you may have felt your definition was acceptable but that patient satisfaction would be too difficult to measure. Still others may have felt that you could not adequately express in words what the term means. As for so many other ideas, concepts, and feelings in our lives, verbal expression is often easier than written expression.

Our definition of patient satisfaction will follow later in this chapter. Even those of us who have spent considerable time thinking about this concept do not believe that we have yet arrived at a totally suitable definition. This uncertainty should be kept in mind as you read this chapter because it suggests that the book is not closed on defining this concept. Please use our ideas as a starting point and improve on them as you see fit. You may conceive of some additional ideas that may improve our understanding of this concept.

Deriving a Global Definition of Patient Satisfaction

Our definition of patient satisfaction is comprised of four ideas. The first three—stimuli, value judgments, and reactions—are described below (Figure 3.1). The fourth idea—individual differences—will be discussed later in this chapter.

Figure 3.1   First Part of Our Definition of Patient Satisfaction

Stimulus	**Patient's Value Judgment**	**Patient's Reaction**
Stethoscope $\longrightarrow$	Cold	$\longrightarrow$ Feels angry toward doctor
40-minute wait $\longrightarrow$	Too long, unacceptable	$\longrightarrow$ Expresses rage at doctor and sends complaint letter
Nurse answers questions $\longrightarrow$	Answers judged as clear and concise	$\longrightarrow$ Compliments nurse and expresses satisfaction
Insurance forms to complete $\longrightarrow$	Hard to read	$\longrightarrow$ Failure to comply and dissatisfied
Doctor walks in with test results $\longrightarrow$	"Fight or flight"	$\longrightarrow$ Heartbeat races

Part I: Stimuli, Value Judgments, and Reactions

Health care organizations are replete with stimuli to which patients may or may not respond. Stimuli are cues in the patients' environment that they may sense, smell, see, feel, or hear. All of the following represent different kinds of stimuli: signs directing patients from one place to another, insurance forms to complete, waivers of liability to sign, the beeping sound on the cardiac monitoring equipment, parking spaces to secure, registration and admitting clerks to work with, decor to notice, hand lotions to smell, the level of comfort of chairs in admitting, physicians' attitudes, nurses' behaviors, laboratory technicians' procedures, and distances to walk. As these stimuli are observed and perceived, patients respond by making conscious or unconscious judgments about them. For example:

- "The registration clerk (stimulus) should lose some weight." (judgment)
- "This form (stimulus) is impossible to understand." (judgment)
- "My room (stimulus) is so spacious (judgment). I love it!" (judgment)
- "I never thought I would be able to rent VCR tapes for my room (stimulus). This is great!" (judgment)

The key to these judgments are the values patients attach to them. Value judgments represent the patients' attempts to assign meaning to the plethora of stimuli to which they are exposed. These value judgments can be expressed in terms such as *good, bad, cold, funny, soft, scary, tasty, helpful, hard to read, positive, negative,* or *neutral.* The value judgments assigned to incoming stimuli represent the first key element of patient satisfaction that we wish to measure.

However, patients do more than make value judgments in response to stimuli. Following the patients' value judgments, patients may (or may not) react (feel and think something more, or do something). They may react affectively and cognitively with feelings and thoughts of satisfaction, dissatisfaction, pleasure, displeasure, anger, joy, or sadness. In addition, patients may react both affectively and behaviorally—for example, the patient is angry (the affect) about a rude nurse and subsequently writes a complaint letter (the behavior). Physiological reaction—-with a faster heart rate, shallow respiration, or profuse perspiration—in our judgment is a form of behavioral reaction.

How do we tell the difference between a "value judgment" and a "reaction"? We suggest that value judgments are essentially efforts on the part of the respondent to evaluatively label stimuli. However, there are instances when value judgments might be viewed as initial reactions to stimuli, as well. This helps to explain why the operational distinction between a value judgment and a reaction may, at times, be blurred.

It is both these value judgments and the patient's subsequent reaction to them that serves as the basis for the first part of our conceptual definition of patient satisfaction:

Part I: Patient satisfaction is conceptually defined as patients' unique value judgments and subsequent reactions to the stimuli that they perceive in the health care environment just before, during, and just after the course of their inpatient stay or clinic visit.

After this buildup, you may have thought that a definition as concise and dramatic as $E = mc^2$ would emerge. However, this definition is as important to those interested in patient satisfaction as $E = mc^2$ is to the physicist. This first part of the definition of patient satisfaction tells health care managers many important things about the patient satisfaction measurement process.

Systematic responses

Patient satisfaction is not a random event because certain stimuli may generate consistent types of value judgments and responses in patients. For instance, if a physician (stimulus) is rushing (value judgment) through office visits with patients, this may be perceived as poor doctor-patient relations skills by the majority of this doctor's patients (related value judgment to "rushing"). Moreover, those who label this as poor doctor-patient relations skills may be more likely to react by changing physicians.

Influence over the patient satisfaction process

We can directly influence patient satisfaction because we can influence the stimuli to which patients are exposed. If we could teach the harried physician to take a little extra time with patients, we would probably see that patients would perceive this doctor more favorably, and thoughts of changing physicians might become less frequent. Not only can we influence value judgments and reactions by directly altering the stimuli, we also can intervene directly at the value judgment stage of the model—for example, by trying to alter the patient's expected value judgments or expectations.

The classic example is the waiting time to get to one's room or see the doctor in a clinic setting. If a patient is left waiting in admitting for four hours without anyone telling her what is causing the delay, then the patient's value judgment about the admitting process is likely to be negative. If, however, an admissions clerk tells the patient that there will be a four-hour wait so the patient has time to run errands instead of waiting in admissions, then the patient's value judgment may tend to be less negative. In this example, the stimulus has remained the same—the patient still has to wait four hours. However, since the admitting clerk provided new information (additional stimuli), the patient's value judgment was altered.

As you may expect, we can also intervene at the reaction stage of this model as well. Suppose a patient is thrashing around and screaming after surgery because he is not permitted to eat solid foods. An explanation of these dietary restrictions might help to calm the patient down. In this example, someone tries to alter the patient's form of expressed reaction by providing additional information (a new stimulus) to allay his displeasure. Service recovery programs are another example of intervening at the reaction stage.

Health care managers probably have the most impact in this model in the actions they can take to alter stimuli and shape value judgments. Intervening at the reaction stage may be more difficult in terms of affecting patient attitudes and behaviors since they occur temporally later in the model.

Perceptual realities

It is the patients' perception of the stimuli that is their reality. These are the "facts" with which health care managers must deal. There is ample research in the fields of cognitive and social psychology to support the contention that people often will misperceive stimuli, leading them to make inaccurate value judgments (Schneider et al. 1979; Nisbett and Ross 1980; Fiske and Taylor 1984). Consequently, their reactions may also appear to be inappropriate or illogical to health care providers and managers. However, from the patients' perspective, this means very little since it is their reality. More specifically, it is their body, their health care experience, and their physical and psychological well-being that is in their mind and heart!

This can be extremely frustrating to the health care manager. A patient might complain that he or she waited too long in x-ray—30 minutes. The manager pleasantly shows the patient recently published national statistics from 2,000 other hospitals in the United States, Canada, and Britain indicating that 30 minutes is among the fastest service times to get in and out of an x-ray in the world! The patient's response is predictable: "That's your opinion. I still waited in a very uncomfortable wheelchair for 30 minutes and that's too long for a medical procedure that takes only milliseconds to perform." The patient's reality is one of many, yet it is still of great importance.

Part II: Individual Differences and Moderating Effects

Part I of our definition focuses on stimuli within the health care environment to which patients make value judgments, leading them to react. Part II of our definition focuses on how our dispositional makeup, personality, need structure, values, beliefs, personal life, and prior health care experiences can modify and shape our responses to these stimuli. To better understand this, consider the following critical incident as it plays out in two hypothetical scenarios involving two distinctly different patients.

The Critical Incident: The phlebotomist was new and inexperienced. At 22 years of age, one could not expect her to have a long lifetime of experience behind her. She had been called to the patient's room to draw some blood. Unfortunately, she had trouble finding a vein. To get enough blood for the lab work, she had to stick two patients four times until she had accumulated a sufficient quantity. She apologized profusely about having to stick the patients so often.

Scenario 1: The first patient is a 34-year-old woman from an affluent, upper-class background. She is in the hospital for a series of tests designed to identify if she is suffering from cardiological problems. She has never been in the hospital before. She is an extremely private person and loathes having to share a room with someone else. She is easy to anger and has little patience. In a conversation with her husband after the blood drawing she said: "I cannot believe this world today. People can't do their jobs properly any more. This technician comes in and can't even find a vein. What kind of medical staff do they have around here? She didn't even say she was sorry!"

Scenario 2: The second patient is a mother of five from an upper middle-class background. She is 41 years old and has been hospitalized seven times previously, six times for obstetrics/gynecological reasons. She cares a great deal about the personal, or "high-touch," time she receives from her doctors and nurses. More than anything else, she needs to trust her medical providers. Roommates don't bother her. She is in the hospital for the same medical reasons as the first patient. After the phlebotomist left, she smiled and said to her husband: "She'll get better over time. It was nice of her to apologize."

Although both patients were presented with the same stimulus (the inexperienced phlebotomist desperately seeking a vein), the women expressed entirely different judgments of care rendered. Why? The people doing the judging (and reacting) were distinctly different people, with different backgrounds, values, and expectations regarding health care. These individual differences influence how the incoming stimuli are interpreted by different patients.

In the above hypothetical scenarios, the first patient's anger, frustration, and lack of experience with health care organizations would not permit her to acknowledge the phlebotomist's apology. The value judgment formed of the phlebotomist was largely negative. The second patient's patience, coupled with her greater experience with health care, differentially shaped the way she interpreted and reacted to the identical stimulus. She discounted the phlebotomist's multiple sticks and focused on her interpersonal skills (the apology). The value judgment she formed was distinctly different, as was her reaction. This example leads us to the second part of our definition of patient satisfaction (Part I is repeated for continuity):

> *Parts I and II*: Patient satisfaction is conceptually defined as patients' value judgments and subsequent reactions to the stimuli they perceive in the health care environment just before, during, and after the course of their inpatient stay or clinic visit. These value judgments and reactions will be influenced by the dispositional characteristics of the patients and their previous life and health care experiences.

For those who think in a linear fashion, it may help to look at Figure 3.2. The message conveyed in Figure 3.2 is that patients make value judgments and react in response to stimuli in the health care environment. Both these value judgments and reactions may be influenced by the personality or disposition of the patient and the experiences he or she has had in life, particularly in health care. For the research methodologists and statisticians among our readers, patients' dispositional and experiential characteristics serve as the moderator variables. Stimuli are the independent variables, value judgments are mediating or intermediate variables, and reactions are dependent variables.

Does the above definition of patient satisfaction mean that if 300 different people were to have the wrong leg amputated, 300 different value

Figure 3.2 A Definition of Patient Satisfaction and the Patient Satisfaction Process

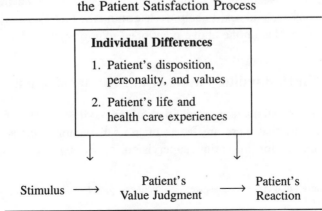

judgments or reactions would emerge of the quality of care received? Although this example is logically taking the concept of individual differences to the *n*th degree, we doubt if 300 different judgments would form. We believe instead that there will be systematic sets of perceptions among different people observing the same set of stimuli. It would be a serious mistake to think that systematic must mean 100 percent similarity among patient perceptions. It may mean as little as 20 percent similarity!

So how is patient satisfaction or dissatisfaction defined within the context of this model? Within the context of the model presented above, patient satisfaction is the patients' reaction in response to stimuli and value judgments as modified by their individual differences. Looking at the model as a whole, patient satisfaction is defined as a dynamic process that involves the relationship between stimuli, value judgments, reactions, and individual differences.

Although patient satisfaction is defined as a process, we do not always measure the complete process within a given survey question. That could be very complex and confusing for both the survey designer and the respondents. Instead, we may choose to measure relationships within the process. For example, we may measure only the presence or absence of the stimulus and extrapolate from that whether or not the patient is satisfied: "In minutes, how long did you wait for the doctor to see you?" If the patient answers 60 minutes or more, we may extrapolate to conclude that this will be dissatisfying. We may also measure the relationship between the stimulus and the value judgment. "The rooms (stimulus) were cold (value judgment). SD D N A SA" or "The nurse (stimulus) listened well (value judgment). SD D N A SA" and again extrapolate how the patient reacted to this.[1] Still other times, we may measure the relationship between the stimulus and the reaction: "I was very satisfied (reaction) with the medical care (stimulus) I received: SD D N A SA." Needless to say, we will also measure sociodemographic factors, such as age and sex, to help us determine the effect (if any) of these moderating variables on the above mentioned relationships.

Understanding Facets of Patient Satisfaction

Facets of patient satisfaction are defined in our model as forms of reaction. In the same way that there are facets of job satisfaction (satisfaction with pay, opportunities for promotion, supervision, co-workers), there are facets

---

1. SD = Strongly Disagree; D = Disagree; N = Neither Agree Nor Disagree; A = Agree; SA = Strongly Agree.

of patient satisfaction, such as satisfaction with physicians, nurses, food, room, environment, parking, and ancillary medical services. Organizing our measurement system around these facets and the stimuli that are likely to affect them can assist us in developing a more useful and valid survey tool. Categorizing these facets and stimuli chronologically from the beginning to the end of the patient's stay will further ensure that the majority of predictable patient stimuli and experiences are covered. Such a list might look as follows:

1. Satisfaction with Preadmission Activities

   Stimuli:

   - Completing forms
   - Communicating with the hospital over the phone
   - Setting up time of admission

2. Satisfaction with Getting to the Hospital

   Stimuli:

   - Accessibility
   - Parking
   - Signs

3. Satisfaction with the Admissions Process and Staff

   Stimuli:

   - Completing forms
   - Waiting time to get to room
   - Attitudes and behaviors of admissions staff
   - Physical environment in the admitting area

4. Satisfaction with the Patient's Room

   Stimuli:

   - Physical environment within the room
   - Comfort
   - Noise levels
   - Lighting
   - Smell
   - Spaciousness
   - Roommate issues
   - Temperature controls

- Cleanliness
- Ease of getting around
- Attitudes and behaviors of housecleaning staff

5. Satisfaction with Food

   Stimuli:

   - Quality of food
   - Temperature of food
   - Choices of food
   - Presentation of food
   - Attitudes and behaviors of dietary staff
   - Smell of the food

6. Environment (Nonroom Issues)

   Stimuli:

   - Hallways
   - X-ray waiting area acceptability
   - Visiting areas
   - Lighting
   - Smell
   - Noise

7. Satisfaction with Medical Care Staff

   A. Satisfaction with Physicians

      Stimuli:

      - Attitudes
      - Behaviors

   B. Satisfaction with Nurses

      Stimuli:

      - Attitudes
      - Behaviors

   C. Satisfaction with Ancillary Medical Staff (Speech Therapy, Lab, etc.)

      Stimuli:

      - Attitudes
      - Behaviors

8. Satisfaction with Personal Physical Factors

Stimuli/value judgments:

- Pain experienced (frequency and intensity)
- Pain management (for example, medication response time)
- Physical comfort during stay
- Handicapped equipment support (for example, rails, bars)

9. Satisfaction with Discharge

Stimuli:

- Forms
- Discharge time
- Home care instructions
- Nursing home arrangements
- Home health care arrangements

10. Satisfaction with Billing

Stimuli:

- Readability and understandability of forms
- Affordability
- Handling of indigent care

11. Satisfaction with Clinical Treatment Aspects of Care

Stimuli/value judgments:

- Procedures conducted painlessly
- Procedures conducted efficiently
- Staff appeared knowledgeable about patient's illness
- Apparent logic of treatment received
- Comfort and pain levels
- Expectation given of course of illness

12. Satisfaction with the Outcomes of Patient's Care

Stimuli/value judgments:

- Better or worse for seeking health care
- Pain levels before and after care
- Psychological outcomes of care—felt safer, more in control, less uncertain
- Quality-of-life measures

This list can, naturally, be expanded to include other stimuli and facets of satisfaction. A key point to remember is that patient satisfaction should be viewed as a multidimensional concept. Our own Patient Satisfaction Measurement System (PSMS) research at Ohio State University and work conducted by Meterko et al. (1990) support this contention.

This does not mean that there is no such thing as overall patient satisfaction. Consumers, in their own minds, are clearly able to express a single and overall evaluation about their health care experiences. However, we believe that the meaning of this overall evaluation may be too varied from patient to patient to generate information that is both useful and reliable. For some patients, the two-hour wait to get in to see their physician may be what is driving their overall feeling of satisfaction or dissatisfaction. For others, it may be the sensitive and caring student nurse who was very attentive during their stay. In other words, "overall satisfaction" to one patient may not mean the same thing as "overall satisfaction" to another. In fact, there could be an infinite number of meanings to the patients' notions of "overall satisfaction." Looking at patient satisfaction as an overall construct, then, may not be nearly as useful, interesting, or reliable to the researcher or manager as looking at various subtypes or facets of patient satisfaction.

The main challenge in patient satisfaction measurement is to define the facets of patient satisfaction and the possible stimuli, value judgments, and dispositional and experiential moderators that influence these reactions. To do this well, the patient satisfaction researcher and the health care manager must allocate a great deal of time and thought to this process. The above-mentioned list of facets of patient satisfaction (and related stimuli/value judgments) may serve as a good starting point in the identification of the concepts you wish to measure.

Back to the Question, What Are We Measuring?

Your specific survey questions should attempt to touch on all aspects of the dynamic model of patient satisfaction present above—stimuli, value judgments, and reactions. Sometimes it will make sense to measure stimuli alone and then correlate the respondents' answers to another question they answer in the survey. For example, in one question you may ask, "How much time did your doctor spend with you during your outpatient visit?" You can then correlate the data from this question with the respondents' answers to the question, "Overall, how satisfied were you with the medical care you received from your doctor?" One might expect that the more time doctors spend with patients, the more satisfied patients will be with the overall care rendered.

Other times it may make sense to link, within the same survey question, a stimulus with a value judgment. For example, you might ask, "The waiting room (stimulus) was comfortable (value judgment). SD D N A SA" An advantage to writing survey items in this way is that it facilitates simplicity—it makes it easy for the respondent to understand the question and answer it. A weakness with this approach is that you cannot necessarily conclude that patients who "strongly agree" or "agree" that the waiting room is comfortable will also be satisfied (the reaction) with the waiting room. For example, it may have been comfortable, but very noisy. Hence, an erroneous conclusion could be drawn.

Still other times, you may choose to measure (and link up) stimuli, value judgments, and reactions all within the same item. For example:

- "It made me feel safe (reaction) when the nurse answered my call light (stimulus) so quickly (value judgment)."
- "The doctor's stethoscope (stimulus) bothered me (reaction) because it was so cold (value judgment)."

The advantage to this approach is that it will generate very specific information about linkages within the model. A weakness is that this approach can result in very lengthy, convoluted, and difficult-to-interpret survey questions.

In sum, you want to capture as many stimuli, value judgments, and facets of satisfaction as possible in the survey you construct. Pay special attention to the kinds of linkages (for example, stimuli linked to value judgments) you are creating in the items you write, and be sure that these are the linkages you are interested in gathering information on. The acid test will be your answer to the following question: Do the linkages I am exploring provide me with information that I am interested in gathering or information that I can actually use to better manage my health care organization? Finally, you will wish to measure moderators—information on the patients' psychosocial dispositions and personal characteristics.

Two Methods for Measuring Patient Satisfaction

Quantitative Methodologies

The quantitative measurement of patient satisfaction is defined as the measurement of patients' stimuli, value judgments, and reactions to their health care experience through numerical representation. Although we have no empirical data for support, we suspect that quantitative methods are the most frequently used methods for measuring patient satisfaction nationwide.

With quantitative methodologies, discharged patients are typically asked a survey question and then given a scale on which they may indicate their responses. The scale may go from Excellent to Poor, Strongly

Disagree to Strongly Agree, or Yes to Maybe to No; numerical values are assigned to each anchor point on the scale. For instance, Excellent might receive the numerical equivalent of a 5, Good might be equivalent to a 4, Average would equal 3, Fair would equal 2, and Poor would equal 1. In its simplest form, quantitative methods might look as shown in Exhibit 3.1 for the fictitious multihospital system, American Health Care, Inc.

Exhibit 3.1   An Example of Quantitative Methods for a Fictitious Multihospital System

---

American Health Care, Inc.
Annual Data for 1991

Responses to the survey question:
"How satisfied were you with your overall hospital stay?"

Response scale:

Very Dissatisfied	Dissatisfied	Neither Satisfied Nor Dissatisfied	Satisfied	Very Satisfied
1 ———————	2 ———————	3 ———————	4 ———————	5

Satisfaction with overall stay, by site

1 = Very Dissatisfied
5 = Very Satisfied

All scores are reported as averages.

	Overall Patient Satisfaction
Health Hospital	4.27
System Hospital 2	4.01
System Hospital 3	3.76
System Hospital 4	3.74
.	
.	
.	
System Hospital 9	2.67

Total system norm = 3.51 $(n = 9)$
   Urban norm   = 3.46 $(n = 6)$
   Suburban norm = 3.61 $(n = 3)$

In this example, we have developed a numerical representation for levels of patient satisfaction with their overall hospital stay. These values are presented for the total sample, for each individual hospital within the system, and for urban and suburban samples.

We first learn that the overall hospital system's absolute score (norm = 3.51) falls between Neither Satisfied Nor Dissatisfied (a value of 3) and Satisfied (a value of 4). We also know that Health Hospital's absolute numerical score is higher than the total sample and that System Hospital 9 is below the norm in absolute value. We use the word "absolute" because these are raw scores and are not yet adjusted for patient age, DRG, and other potentially important moderating factors. In sum, quantitative survey methods allow patients to respond to survey questions with some sort of numerical representation for their value judgments and reactions to their health care stimuli. Chapter 6 focuses on how to develop quantitative survey items.

Qualitative Methods

In qualitative measurement, the health care manager is collecting information by asking patients to write or to express verbally (as in interviews and focus groups) their view of stimuli and their value judgments and reactions to these. The kinds of questions that elicit qualitative data from patients vary. For instance, patients may be asked to write about their impression of how well or poorly their physicians and nurses communicated with them. In other cases, patients may be asked to identify two aspects of their stay that they liked the best and two they liked the least. Many surveys simply leave space at the end for "other" or "general comments."

A key issue with qualitative methods is the analysis of these written or verbal comments. Elaborate and systematic coding mechanisms to analyze qualitative data can be developed, permitting the categorization and subsequent sorting of qualitative data. For example, in Ohio State University's Patient Satisfaction Measurement System, all the written comments about physicians, nurses, admitting, dietary, clinical treatment, ancillary health care staff, and so on are broken down into specific categories. These comments are then further sorted as to whether the patient's value judgment was positive, neutral, or negative. These categories are further broken down by type of positive or negative comment—for example, comments about physician communication skills, comments about the amount of time physicians spent with their patients, and comments about how caring the physicians appeared to be. Finally, these written comments, after being entered into a data base, are re-sorted by nursing discharge unit, medical service, and other variables decided upon by management. An example of Patient Satisfaction Measurement System's qualitative analysis scheme is presented in Chapter 9.

Quantitative or numerical techniques can be applied to qualitative analysis, and we strongly encourage this as long as the inherent associated statistical problems are understood and controlled for. For example, the ratio of positive to negative comments for a given category (for example, dietary) may be monitored on a monthly basis and then trended over time.

Often, qualitative data can be more useful than quantitative data. There are a few reasons for this. First, patients may feel less constrained when not confined to a multiple-choice format. Quantitative survey items may not be phrased or worded in ways that the patient understands and can relate to. What is more, the limitations imposed by any quantitative response scale may fail to represent the depth and intensity of an individual patient's health care experience. Qualitative comments often allow patients to say exactly what they feel in their own words.

Second, patients may be more willing to offer negative feedback through their qualitative comments. Many times we have read patient surveys where the patient quantitatively indicates high levels of satisfaction with his or her experience, and yet the same patient's qualitative comments address many areas in which the patient was dissatisfied. This situation may occur because the qualitative survey questions permit patients to express their value judgments and reactions with the added precision of context— for example, "I know the nurses were trying their hardest and were very busy, but they were consistently late with my medications and that made me very mad!" From the patients' perspective, qualitative survey questions may allow them to explain exactly how they feel and why they feel that way, sometimes, buffering a negative comment by presenting it in light of some context, as noted in the above example.

Conclusion

What we are trying to measure is a process linking stimuli to patient value judgments to patient reactions and moderated by individual differences. The specific concept of patient satisfaction, some may argue, is embedded in patient reactions; however, the process of patient satisfaction, involving stimuli, value judgments, and individual differences, must not be forgotten. It is this process that we must uncover and learn about, not just the end reaction of patients feeling satisfied or dissatisfied. It is insufficient for the researcher and health care manager to ask simply about levels of satisfaction with various facets of health care, such as asking patients to rate their satisfaction with waiting times, food, their doctor, and nursing care on a scale from 1 to 5. The challenge to measuring patient satisfaction is in identifying what patients are thinking and feeling and why they think and feel this way: the causal process. The quantitative and qualitative methodologies we briefly outlined in this chapter represent two broad approaches to attaining this end. Part III of this book discusses these methodologies in depth.

4

LEARNING ABOUT THE POPULATION
WE WISH TO SURVEY

In this chapter, we will discuss why it is so important to learn as much as possible about the survey population. In addition, we will offer you specific methodologies on how this can be accomplished.

Learning about our survey population is not as easy to accomplish as one may initially think. There are many different kinds of patients we wish to survey, and to complicate matters sometimes their family and friends are the ones who actually respond to the patient satisfaction surveys.

Why Learn about Respondents?

Understanding the clinical and demographic dimensions of the population we are surveying is crucial for effective patient satisfaction measurement for a variety of reasons.

Research Control and Precision

The more knowledge we have of the population of patients we survey, the more precise and accurate our patient satisfaction survey research conclusions will be. Consider the following example to better understand this point.

The Health Care System for the Self-Important and Wealthy has two hospitals. Noteworthy is that one of the hospitals, Gold Memorial, serves older patients than the other hospital, the Emerald Foundation Hospital. Overall satisfaction with one's hospital stay on a ten-point scale is 9.32 for Gold, but only 8.43 for Emerald.

Our normal inclination would be to conclude immediately that Gold has higher patient satisfaction performance than Emerald—after all its score for patient satisfaction with overall stay is higher. However, such a conclusion could be erroneous.

What if the two different satisfaction scores could be attributed to something other than better or worse job performance—something like patient age? Specifically, consider the fact that older patients express higher levels of satisfaction with their overall inpatient stay than younger patients. We have observed this in one of our PSMS sites, and Meterko et al. (1990, p. S41) found a similar relationship among 710 discharged inpatients they surveyed. Now suppose, as noted above, that Gold serves a much larger proportion of older patients than Emerald. If this is the case, then the difference in scores could be due to the different age of the patient populations each hospital serves! That is, the satisfaction scores for Emerald may be lower because it is treating younger patients, who are perhaps more difficult to satisfy.

Now the most important point of all: If we did not have accurate information on patient age, the erroneous conclusion that Gold is "better" (in some way) than Emerald could be drawn all too easily.

Being Able to Generalize

Unless we understand the demographic and clinical composition of our total population of discharges and those who do not respond to the survey, we cannot meaningfully generalize our results. If we do not know that the majority of the people who respond to our survey are patients 54 years and older, then the data generated by this group may be inappropriately generalized to younger patients. In Chapter 7, methods of assessing the generalizability of your survey results are discussed in depth.

Targeting Successful Solutions

Similarly, we cannot target our solutions in response to service or clinical problem areas that patients identify unless we again have a relatively complete understanding of the patient population we serve. If 95 percent of our survey respondents are women, and we are *unaware* of this, then a given solution to a problem cited by this sample may actually hurt a large portion of our patient population (the males) who did not respond to the survey. Hence, employing the wrong (or nongeneralizable) intervention to solve a problem could actually do more harm than good. This, obviously, must be avoided at all costs.

The above leads us to conclude that we have no choice but to learn as much about our respondents and patient population as possible! Otherwise, patient satisfaction measurement will become less meaningful and more risky. How can we accomplish this?

The Logic of Encoding

The PSMS research project has begun to show that a promising way to generate accurate clinical and demographic information on both respondents and nonrespondents is by encoding patient names, and other pertinent demographic and clinical information regarding their stay, onto each individual survey prior to distribution. Though we were originally concerned that this practice might decrease our survey return rate, we have found that, basically, the same (or a higher percentage) of surveys are returned, whether the survey is preencoded or not. Reminder letters were not sent to nonrespondents.

Our research shows that when given the opportunity to voluntarily sign surveys that are not preencoded, 82 percent of our respondents do (PSMS data, 1989–1990, four-month sampling of over 1,750 returned surveys). When patient names are encoded on surveys and subsequently mailed to them, our research shows that the return rate is the same as when patients are given the option of supplying their names on surveys that are not preencoded.

This observation implies that the patients who respond are typically people who are willing to use their names. If they are willing to use their names, then they may be less concerned about having other information about themselves and their health care experience encoded on the survey before mailing. If this can be done, then it is possible to gather a great deal of accurate demographic and clinical information about the patients who do and do not respond.

Asking patients to report information about themselves and their stay is not recommended. Patients, due to a host of factors—for example, acuity, age, anxiety, size of hospital, medications, personality—are known to supply inaccurate information about themselves and their stay. For instance, many PSMS respondents demonstrate that they have enormous difficulty remembering what room number and what medical building they were in—especially if they were transferred within the hospital during their stay. For other patients, their physician's name may be a blur because "there were so many of them."

This is not to belittle our patients—most of us would have the same difficulty if we were surveyed following a hospitalization. Rather, we must recognize that the nature of a health care encounter makes it very difficult for patients to accurately report data about themselves and their stay to the patient satisfaction researcher.

Our second conclusion is, Do not rely on patients to accurately report objective information on certain aspects of their stay, such as length, location, medical condition, and attending physician. Instead, it may make a lot more sense to rely on an encoding methodology.

The Specifics of Encoding

By "encoding," we mean placing information from the patient's medical record onto each patient's individual survey via a mailing label or direct printing on the survey itself.

What kind of information is crucial? We recommend the following, though this list could easily be altered or expanded to fit your health care organization's particular needs:

1. Patient's name

2. Address

3. Phone number

4. DRG number

5. Medical service

6. Attending or admitting physician

7. Nursing discharge unit

8. Length of stay

9. Medical record number

10. Sex

11. Age

12. Acuity measures (if available)

13. Medical diagnostic classification

14. ICD-9 code

15. Payer source.

Figure 4.1 is a sample of a PSMS encoded mailing label. It is an adhesive label that is affixed to the survey itself. Hospitals and outpatient clinics with whom we work extract information from each patient's medical record and place it onto a larger mailing label.

When the surveys are returned, the patient satisfaction survey researcher and health care manager have attained the key goal of now knowing as much as possible about the respondents. As importantly, this information

Figure 4.1 Sample of PSMS Mailing Label

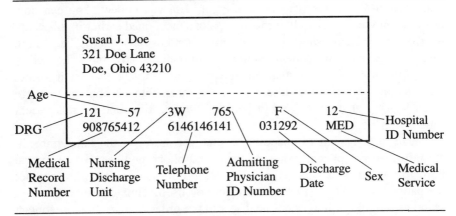

Note: Information below the broken line does not appear in the envelope window. Masked codes are also an option.

will be accurate since it is based, not on the patient's self-report for these nonperceptual variables, but on information taken directly from the patient's medical record.

The Research and Analytical Advantages to Encoding

In light of our earlier discussion on why we must learn about the population of patients we serve, look again at the research and analytical advantages of encoding.

Suppose you know that 15 percent of all your hospital's discharges are from your obstetrics service. However, you note that in your sample of respondents, you have received only 4 percent from this service. This should warn you that there may be some uneven representation in your sample and that you should be very careful about how you interpret your data.

Another benefit to encoding is that by learning about your respondents you will also be learning about your nonrespondents, assuming that your health care organization can provide equally detailed information about the total population it serves. Your organization may have these data via previous market research, census by service studies, or patient utilization and origin studies. For example, suppose you find that your response sample underrepresents oncology discharges for patients 60 years and older. This may tell you that your survey methods are not appropriate for older oncology patients, or that perhaps there is something within your survey that inhibits your older oncology patients from responding (for example, the survey's length).

A third benefit to encoding is that it expands your analytical and re-search control over the patient satisfaction data you collect: You can now break down your data by all of the dimensions mentioned earlier in this chap-ter (for example, nursing discharge unit, attending physician). The health care manager and the patient satisfaction researcher now have the ability to *account for* the results that emerge from the survey; that is, it allows them to answer questions like, "Have we taken into account patient age when looking at the relationship between waiting time and overall patient satisfaction?"

A fourth benefit to encoding is that you have on the label immedi-ate information—patient name, address, and phone number. Hence, if you must follow up on a satisfaction survey, the information needed to contact the patient is readily available on the survey itself. Time-consuming record searches through billing or medical records in order to learn how to contact the patient become unnecessary.

In sum, knowing who your respondent is dramatically enhances your level of research and managerial control. It allows you to recognize many important aspects of the patient's demographic background and medical con-dition that may account for the level of patient satisfaction reported in your data. Encoding surveys adds an enormous amount of control to the patient satisfaction measurement process.

Potential Problems with Encoding

One potential concern is whether the respondent will delete the encoded information or tear off the label. Although we originally were concerned that respondents might do this, we have found in our field trials and subsequently that only 1–2 percent of 3,000 returned surveys had the encoded information erased or deleted by the respondent.

A second concern, as discussed earlier, is a lower response rate. Our fear was that encoded labels would make the respondent feel too identifi-able and hence threatened. Our field trials (and subsequent work) show no decrement in response rate due to encoding.

A third concern is enhanced leniency effects; that is, respondents, be-cause of their concern over being identified, may be frightened of being critical of the health care organization and its providers. Again, our early results do not indicate that this is a problem, though more data need to be collected. Noteworthy is that the patients' qualitative comments are no less critical when encoding is employed.

A fourth concern is the delay in sending out surveys due to the time needed to encode the survey. We have found with our sites that within two to seven days of discharge most, if not all, the information you need to place on the encoded label/survey is available. However, this may not be true in some hospitals where medical records systems are less automated.

A fifth concern is one of confidentiality. Since the encoded information, for the most part, is a string of numbers and letters that could mean almost anything, the patient's confidentiality seems intact. Numbers and letters (the codes) can be easily disguised via substitute and masked codes as well. (For instance, the medical service code "MED" could be masked as "YYY" on the label.) Moreover, the codes can be placed on the survey in a way that minimizes the likelihood of anyone but the patient seeing them.

A sixth concern is creating accurate matches between the content of the survey and the information encoded on the label. Consider a patient who was in intensive care and then moved elsewhere in the hospital prior to discharge. If the encoded label only lists this patient's nursing discharge unit, then to which group are this patient's nursing evaluations from the survey referring to? Intensive care nurses, the nursing discharge unit nurses, or both?

There are two ways to handle this. One way is to encode on the label if the patient has been transferred during his or her stay, and then break this group out of your statistical analysis. The second method is to have separate sections of the survey that refer to nursing care in ICU (if applicable) and nursing care in the unit the patient was discharged from.

Note that the same problem can occur with encoded physician identification numbers. How can we be sure that the physician the patient is referring to in the survey is the same physician encoded on the label? Naturally, we could ask patients to supply the name of the physician they are referring to in their survey responses; however, this approach has problems too. This problem is, perhaps, even larger than the accurate identification of nurses, and it is discussed in depth in the next chapter.

While the encoded label offers many advantages, there are difficulties with using it that must be considered as well. As a result, we do not wish to oversell our preliminary success with encoding. Clearly, our experience with it is still too new and limited to draw any absolute conclusions, and much more study is needed. The early returns, however, suggest that encoding is a promising way to answer the key question this chapter poses: Who are we surveying?

"I Thought Only Patients Completed Patient Satisfaction Surveys?"

One of the nastiest surprises in patient satisfaction measurement is to learn that patients are not the only ones completing the surveys. For example, sometimes the patient is too ill to complete the survey, and his or her family member or friend will read the items and record the patient's response. This poses no serious problem.

What does pose a serious problem is when nonpatients start answering survey questions from their own views, rather than the patient's, putting us back into the same old mess: Who are we surveying?

Originally, we believed we could finesse this problem by asking the following question as the first question on the survey:

Who is filling out this survey?
1. Patient
2. Other (e.g., family member, friend, etc.)

Asking this question, we thought, would allow the evaluator to get a more precise measure of who is responding. With this information, the patient satisfaction researcher is now able to run an analysis separating "patient" responses from those of the "other" group. One can now measure how the "patient" group perceives the health care experience and how the "other" group perceives the experience.

In analyzing our PSMS data, we have found that the "other" group is typically less satisfied than the "patient" group across a variety of satisfaction indicators; that is, the patient's spouse, parents, and friends—those "others" filling out the survey for the patient (or themselves)—are less satisfied with the patient's overall hospital stay than the "patient" group ($t = 2.99$; $p \leq$ .003, 191.22 degrees of freedom). This might suggest that not only must we work hard to make our patients satisfied, but we must do the same with the closely orbiting satellite of family and friends surrounding the patient. However, this statistically significant difference could be accounted for by other factors, such as the patient's acuity and length of stay.

The problem with this methodology is that we asked the wrong question (what's new?)! The reason lies in a probable methodological confound within the "other" group. This group's responses are most probably comprised both of those family members and friends who are recording the patient's value judgments and reactions (which is fine) and of those family and friends recording their own views of the patient's health care experience, not the patient's (which is not fine)! The issue has less to do with who is filling out the survey, and more to do with whose value judgments and reactions are expressed in the survey. We are not suggesting that the perceptions of family members or others should be discounted or that they are not worth evaluating, but they do confound the information collected.

Because family members and others are participants in the hospital experience and the postdischarge care of the patient, one potential avenue to pursue to help reduce this confound in information is to design and provide a separate survey to the family members and others. In this way, you can clearly state to them that it is their perceptions and viewpoints in which you are interested.

In light of this confound we have begun to rely on a second methodology, developed by a PSMS team member, which we believe is better. The last question of the survey should read:

Whose viewpoints are expressed in this survey?
1. Patient
2. Other (e.g., family, friend, or spouse)

This allows health care managers to be more secure in knowing whether they are measuring the value judgments and reactions of the patient or someone else. The result is exactly what we are trying to accomplish: We now have a much better idea of whom we are measuring. When we conduct the analysis, we can now separate the two groups and, in doing so, remove the confound.

Conclusion

State-of-the-art patient satisfaction measurement requires us to know as much about our respondents and nonrespondents as possible. To draw meaningful, useful, and circumspect conclusions from patient satisfaction feedback, we have to know who is doing the writing and whose points of view are being expressed. Encoding surveys and identifying who is the source of the information provided in a survey are two key steps in this direction. It significantly increases the power of the tool for both quantitative and qualitative patient satisfaction measurement and subsequent managerial applications.

PART III

HOW TO MEASURE
PATIENT SATISFACTION

5

THE LAYOUT AND DESIGN
OF THE SURVEY

Tempting as it may be, the next step is not to start writing survey questions. There is a major antecedent step that still needs to be accomplished. You need to develop a conceptual framework for your survey. This involves creating an organizational structure for your survey, which is the first major issue we address in this chapter. Following, we will provide some guidelines to help you get the respondent started in completing the survey.

Level One: Macrolevel Design

There are many possibilities for macrolevel design and they are not mutually exclusive. One method is to create sections of the survey that are organized around different provider facets of patient satisfaction. For instance, the first section might be called "Satisfaction with Your Physician's Care"; the second section, "Satisfaction with Your Nursing Care"; the third section, "Satisfaction with Your Room"; and so on. In the survey systems we have implemented, many rely, at least in part, on this design strategy.

A second option would be to focus on "critical incidents," important events (stimuli) that patients typically encounter during their hospital stay. For instance, the first section might be called "Your Admission"; the second section, "Learning about Your Health Care Problem"; and the third, "Interactions with Nonmedical Staff."

A third method, and the one that we recommend, is actually a hybrid of the first two: It includes both facets of satisfaction and critical incidents (stimuli). However, these are organized within one overall chronological framework, beginning with preadmission and ending with billing. Sections might be presented in the following order:

1. Preadmission
2. Admission
3. Room
4. Food
5. Environment
6. Physician care
7. Nursing care
8. Clinical treatment
9. Radiological technicians, laboratory staff, and other members of the medical professional care team
10. Discharge planning
11. Discharge
12. Patient's medical outcomes
13. Postdischarge
14. Billing

We suggest this method for at least two reasons. First, it is relatively consistent with patients' temporal experiences in either the hospital or outpatient setting. It is easy for most patients to follow this sequence because they are encouraged to begin their cognitive process chronologically at one point in time and end at another, giving "phenomenological validity" to the organization of the survey; that is, through this method, we are measuring patients' responses to stimuli in the order in which the phenomena are likely to have occurred.

Second, this method may actually help patients recall information about their stay. It is logical that patients are more likely to accurately and comprehensively reconstruct their health care experiences if we provide them with a chronological outline of the sequence of events they were likely to have undergone. The phrase "Go ahead and tell me your story, from the beginning," often used by police officers working with distraught crime victims, may be a cognitive structure that has informally emerged over time in order to aid us in recalling information accurately and comprehensively.

Level Two: Microlevel Design

How do we organize survey questions that will comprise these broad, macrolevel categories? There are a few guidelines we suggest.

Rule 1: Use Chronological Order

The order of questions within each macrolevel section should follow the chronology of the patient's stay. For example, consider preadmission: A question about ease of filling out preadmission forms mailed to the patient's home would come before a question about parking because the former event temporally precedes the latter.

Rule 2: Specific Judgments Should Precede More Global Judgments

Patients should be asked to respond to questions about specific component parts of their stay or visit prior to being asked to make a global judgment of their overall stay or clinic visit. For example, suppose we have four specific survey questions in our "Nursing Care" macrolevel section:

My nurses at Health Hospital were

Pleasant	SD	D	N	A	SA
Responsive	SD	D	N	A	SA
Courteous	SD	D	N	A	SA
Communicative	SD	D	N	A	SA

In addition, there is a fifth "global" question:

Overall, how satisfied were you with the quality of the nursing care you received at Health Hospital?

| Extremely Dissatisfied | | | | | | Extremely Satisfied |
| 1 | 2 | 3 | 4 | 5 | 6 | 7 |

Now, the question we are facing becomes one of ordering. Should the global question be presented first or last within the "Nursing Care" macrolevel section?

Our first choice, putting the global question last, represents a specific——→global approach. It is logical that respondents should answer specific items about their health care experience before being asked about their overall (or more global) feelings. This order allows patients to form a more global perspective on their level of satisfaction based on the specific survey items leading up to the global question. The flaw with this argument is that the survey researcher may be limiting the thought that goes into the respondent's "global" impression to exclusively the antecedent survey questions. Hence, although the patient may personally think that the primary nurse had an "upbeat" attitude, the patient may fail to report this because he or she is focusing only on the survey items provided and not on "attitude."

It is this flaw that serves as the best argument in favor of asking the global item first, and the micro items second: global——→specific. The flaw with the global——→specific approach is one of "cognitive consistency"— the respondent's desire to be consistent in how he or she answers survey questions and perceives the world in general (Bem 1967; Festinger 1957). Hence, if the respondent answers Extremely Satisfied to the global item, he or she will be predisposed to answer Extremely Satisfied to the specific items that follow. Most respondents want to perceive themselves as consistent in their thought patterns, attitudes, and behaviors, as well as to have others perceive them in the same way.

Is this a catch–22 or is there a way out? The answer is that there is no perfect solution, but the flaw of the specific——→global approach seems less fatal than the flaw of the global——→specific approach. If patient satisfaction researchers do their homework and include a comprehensive list of specific survey items, then it may be safer to present these specific items first, and the global item second. Moreover, if open-ended questions are provided, the potential risk of not being comprehensive in covering the totality of the patient's experience is somewhat mitigated (see Chapter 9, on qualitative patient satisfaction measurement.)

By now you may be wondering, "When will we start putting together an actual patient satisfaction survey? Enough of this background material already!" In actuality, we have been building your survey all along. You now know some key elements in designing an effective patient satisfaction measurement system. We have discussed the costs and benefits of patient satisfaction measurement (Chapters 1 and 2), what you are trying to measure (Chapter 3), who you are measuring (Chapter 4), and how your survey should be organized along both macro and micro dimensions (Chapter 5).

Rule 3: Include Space for Qualitative Comments

One reason for including space for qualitative comments at the end of each macrolevel section is that the respondent is already thinking about the topical theme of a given macrolevel section after filling out the preceding specific and global items. Asking respondents to come back to the same theme later in the survey is less efficient; hence, respondents may be less willing to offer their qualitative value judgments and reactions. Moreover, the specific items preceding the space allocated for written comments may help to trigger pertinent qualitative comments. If this occurs, you want to make it easy for the respondent to immediately record this information on the survey.

The foundation for effective patient satisfaction measurement is almost built. In the next section of this chapter, we will add the finishing touches by discussing the introductory and instructive sections of your survey and their implications for response rates, marketing, and generating valid and reliable data. Then we will move on to designing specific survey questions in Chapter 6.

Getting the Respondent Started: The Survey Front Matter, Instructions, and Ethics

Many people mistakenly believe that the patient satisfaction survey begins with the survey itself; however, the survey actually begins with the envelope the patient receives in the mail.

The Envelope

What does the patient satisfaction researcher wish to accomplish through the envelope in which the survey is distributed? First, the researcher does not want to breach the patient's confidentiality. Suppose the envelope has typed on it in its lower left-hand corner in red letters: "Inpatient Satisfaction Survey Enclosed." From the patient's perspective, this could be construed as a breach of confidentiality. For example, a college student living with roommates might not want it known that he or she entered the hospital for a day of psychiatric testing. Similarly, a mother of a teenager might not want her daughter to know about a biopsy she underwent until she gets the results and is able to assimilate them herself. The patient is entitled to privacy. As in most areas of health care, when conducting patient satisfaction surveys, we must remember that ethics, including protecting patient confidentiality and anonymity, precedes all.

At the same time, patient satisfaction researchers want to maximize the response rate. Specifically, they want to encourage the addressee to open the envelope and not throw it out with the junk mail. Hence, placing nothing on the envelope may be risky, though for a different reason. Here are some guidelines to help you resolve this problem.

1. Do not identify the contents of the envelope on the envelope itself.

2. Place the hospital's logo and return address on the envelope.

3. If you feel compelled, you can print on the front of the envelope something such as "Important information enclosed" or "Please open—we need to know what you think." (This could even be risky because it takes a step closer to revealing the envelope's contents.) These messages encourage the person to open the envelope, yet they do not reveal the contents. From the above language, the envelope could contain marketing materials, an invitation to the opening of

a new medical building, an outstanding bill, or reconfirmation of insurance payment.

4. Avoid putting anything too "cutesy" or "gimmicky" on the envelope:

   • "Win a free VCR. Details inside."

   • "Nothing to fear. Open it here!"

   • "Win a round-trip ticket for two to Europe. Details inside."

   • "Bulletin, Bulletin . . ."

   • "TWOFERS—Two for one cardiac catheterizations. Details inside and no obligation."

If you actually do have these incentives for filling out the survey, as discussed in Chapter 7, you may get patients completing the survey in a haphazard fashion (for example, circling all 5s) just so they can qualify for the prize or allay their guilt for taking the "enclosed pen," thus compromising the validity of your survey data. In a randomized trial conducted by Meterko et al. (1990), including a pen with the survey increased response rates by 10 percent ($p < .05$). As tempting as this may be, we believe the risk of generating haphazard results is not worth the increased response rate incentives may bring.

Introducing the Survey

Assume that the discharged patient has received the envelope and opened it up. Now what? All front matter to the actual survey itself—attached cover letter, letter on the first page of the survey, instructional materials—should be designed with the following goals in mind.

Goal 1: Protect confidentiality and anonymity

Respondents must get the message that their confidentiality and anonymity are fully protected. This should be stated simply and directly on the survey. Tell patients clearly who will be reviewing their individual survey, informing respondents that their doctor will not see any negative comments they may write. Also state that their responses to the survey will be grouped with others, so that no one will be able to identify individual responses or comments. In addition, you may wish to note that qualitative comments that could identify the source will be edited. We cannot emphasize enough the importance of including these statements. You are in jeopardy of collecting invalid and unreliable data if respondents feel that you may show their survey to their health care providers. The reassurance of confidentiality and anonymity is required for ethical reasons, as well as for practicing good research methods.

But exactly how far should you go in reassuring the respondents? For example, should the front matter to the survey specifically state, "You may detach the encoded mailing label if you choose," or "No doctors will ever see your individual survey. We promise"? If you go overboard in reassuring people, you may actually increase the chances of stirring up respondent anxiety. Our best advice is to reassure them as much as you feel ethically and legally obligated. A basic and clearly stated assurance of confidentiality and anonymity alone should be sufficient. Ultimately, however, this is an individual judgment call for the patient satisfaction researcher, the health care organization's attorney, and the manager.

Goal 2: Encourage honest responses

Most patient satisfaction researchers would agree that there is a positive response set bias in how respondents fill out patient satisfaction surveys. Sometimes called a *leniency effect*, respondents seem to be easy graders when exposed to quantitative methodologies. Why?

One explanation is that they are simply telling us the truth, and they are not really easy graders. Since the vast majority of outcomes from inpatient stays are positive (that is, the patient gets well or is made to feel better), the dissatisfying effects of cold food, waiting too long for pain medications, and slow nurse response times may be psychologically discounted by the patient when completing the survey. We certainly know that patients are capable of being brutally negative. Moreover, it is interesting to note that we are more likely to find negative opinions reflected in a written qualitative comment than in a numerical quantitative representation of how the patient feels. We have often found that the patient grades the overall experience a 9 or 10 (the best), but then writes in many negative comments.

Another explanation is that the quantitative methods may unintentionally encourage leniency. Some of the survey questions may be leading: "Didn't you think your physician care was absolutely wonderful? SD D N A SA." Also, the hospital may only be asking questions about critical incidents (stimuli) they know they will score well on: "Did the TV in your room work?" or "Were there sufficient visiting hours for family and friends?" or "Did you see a nurse at least once?"

Finally, as previously discussed, respondents may be frightened of criticizing their health care providers. They may fear that when they need health care in the future, their doctor may treat them differently due to their responses to the survey.

A good way to encourage sincere answers from your respondents is through a paragraph such as the following:

We at Health Hospital need to hear about the things you liked and did not like about your hospital stay. There are no right or wrong answers, so we encourage your honest response.

Goal 3: Encourage your respondents to complete the survey

What is said up front may influence response rates. Obviously, guaranteeing confidentiality and anonymity is a step in the right direction, as is requesting honest responses. However, there is more you can do.

First, tell your respondents in the introductory material why their participation is so vitally important. Here are some arguments you might use:

1. Your participation in this survey will help us to improve our services.
2. Your feedback will help you and other Health Hospital patients in the future.
3. We want to deliver the best services and quality of care possible. We are not able to do this unless you tell us how you feel about your visit to the Health Clinic.

Second, tell respondents that they do not have to complete every single item on the survey:

Although we want you to complete the entire survey, please leave blank those questions that do not apply to you or that you wish not to complete.

Some people believe that if they cannot complete the whole survey, they should not fill out any of it. Since any valid data you can gather from even just one respondent increases the quality of your data base, nothing could be further from the truth.

Third, tell the respondents that every returned survey will be read. Some surveys even have an item that asks, "Would you like a person from our patient representative's office to call you?" Many patients we telephone are astonished that someone took the time and personal interest to actually read through their entire survey.

Fourth, make the instructions regarding how to fill out the survey simple. "Simple" means not only clear and understandable, but easy to read and comprehend. Short sentences with a single thought are recommended.

Please circle the number that best expresses how you feel. If a question does not apply to you, then please **leave it blank**. Although you may skip questions, try to complete as much of the survey as possible. There are no right or wrong answers, so please tell us how you honestly feel. Again, your confidentiality and anonymity are guaranteed.

Fifth, use pedagogical tools, such as **bold face**, *italics*, underlining, asterisks, numbers, letter spacing, and alternate fonts and type sizes liberally, visually and psychologically differentiating the text for the reader and making the introductory material more readable. This also helps to draw the respondent's attention to particular issues. In contrast, it would be a mistake to give the patient two hundred words of introductory information in a single block paragraph written in tiny letters. Also, use a type size that is as large as possible. Many of your respondents are older and may have less than 20/20 vision.

Sixth, if you are using an encoded label, explain to the respondent that the information on the label is to help the hospital to better analyze and use the information collected. Explaining its presence on the survey should prevent the respondent from tearing it off.

Goal 4: Develop introductory material with marketing in mind

Every interaction with a patient should be seen as a potential marketing opportunity. This is true for the patient satisfaction survey and the front matter contained therein. Some hospitals and clinics may find it useful to state on the cover of their survey: "Please confidentially communicate with us," or "Help us make a difference." There are marketing implications to these statements. The first sends the message that your hospital wants to communicate personally and confidentially with its discharged patients. The second sends the message that your hospital seriously considers what its consumers have to say. It is important to recognize that you are talking to consumers throughout all aspects of your survey, including the introductory materials. How you will be heard, interpreted, and ultimately judged can have significant marketing consequences.

In this front matter, it is equally important that your graphic design, including layout, color, typeface, symbols, and logo, presents an attractive and inviting appearance. The quality of paper on which the survey is printed also conveys to your patients how important the survey process is and what is going to be done with the information in the future. Health care organizations must be careful not to unwittingly send subtle negative messages to their patients by the way the survey looks, feels, and reads.

Placement of the Front Matter

Explanations of the survey's purpose, instructions on completing it, and expressions of appreciation for participating can be located in a variety of places. One choice is to include a cover letter with the survey. Addressed to a general respondent (for example, "Dear Patient") and signed by the CEO, the manager of patient relations, or both, the cover letter can be used as a medium to include much of the above information. PSMS has used this approach over the past two years with success. We believe a letter signed by the hospital's CEO adds a level of credibility and legitimacy to the survey process. Of course, a cover letter will be more costly to your program. As you might expect, the base printing costs for a large hospital with, for example, 20,000 discharges per year, would be substantial. Use of the hospital's letterhead stationery and the weight the letter adds to the outbound mail increase costs. For outpatient surveys sampling populations of varying sizes, added costs will occur, as well.

A second and more frugal choice is to include the front matter information on the inside cover of the survey itself. Although this is a perfectly acceptable alternative, there is at least one drawback—you are decreasing the space for survey items. Moreover, a survey in the mail without a cover letter preceding it may seem less personal and professional. Hence, our recommendation is to use a cover letter if you can afford it. Use the survey itself to reiterate points about the survey system that you wish to stress, such as protection of confidentiality and how to use the response scales.

At the end of the chapter are a few examples of cover letters, instructional text, and introductions. These samples are to be used as guidelines only, since you will want to tailor your survey to your health care organization's unique needs.

Conclusion

We cannot stress enough the importance of sound survey design and organization. In addition, the sequencing of major sections, and specific items and global items, should be given careful consideration. In the pretest of your survey instrument, you should make a point of asking respondents whether they found the survey's framework helpful, user-friendly, and logical, and whether it allowed them to give useful information.

Similarly, how you get the patient started on the survey itself is important. If you did not realize it before you should realize it now: *Little things mean a lot!* Envelope design and the way you word instructions can make a difference in the success of your system.

Finally, the guidelines offered in this chapter are not meant to hem you in and limit your options. We do not have access to the universe of information on these issues. You may have very acceptable, if not better, alternatives to some of our ideas. Moreover, your health care organization, the population it serves, and general situation may differ. If you have found a better way, drop us a note and tell us what it is.

It is now time to start writing specific and global items for your patient survey system.

Exhibit 5.1 Sample Cover Letter

TO THE PATIENTS OF GET WELL COMMUNITY HOSPITAL

The physicians, nurses, and staff of Get Well Community Hospital would like to thank you for using our services and giving us the opportunity to help you during this important time in your life.

In order to continue to be responsive to your needs and those of future patients, we would appreciate you taking a few moments to comment upon your stay by completing the enclosed survey. We assure you that all of the information contained within the survey is *confidential*, and it will not be associated with your name in any public setting.

Please share your thoughts about your hospital stay with us. Your opinion is highly valued by us, and it will greatly help each of us in improving our care and services. I thank you for your help.

Sincerely,

John Doe
Executive Director and President
Get Well Community Hospital

Enclosure

Exhibit 5.2 Sample Instructions

DIRECTIONS:

Please respond to each question by checking the box that best describes your experience during your most recent stay at Get Well Community Hospital. If a question or set of questions are not applicable to this stay, please leave it blank.

Exhibit 5.3   Sample Introductory Letter for Survey or Separate Mailing

MAKE A DIFFERENCE BY LETTING US KNOW HOW WE DID

We at the Get Well Outpatient Clinic want to know about your recent outpatient visit. Your confidential evaluation and suggestions help us improve our services and make the outpatient experience better for our future patients. The label on your survey allows us to better analyze the responses from all of our patients.

Please take a few moments to answer the questions that follow. Then, fold the survey so that the return address and prepaid postage appear on the outside, and drop it in the mail.

Thank you for giving us the opportunity to serve you, and for helping us better meet the needs of our patients and their families.

Mary Doe, C.P.A.
Chief Operating Officer
Get Well Outpatient Clinic

Exhibit 5.4   Sample Introduction to Survey or Cover Letter

PLEASE HELP US MAKE A DIFFERENCE

We would like you to comment on your MOST RECENT visit to the Get Well Clinic.

Your participation in this survey is important. Your candid responses will help us evaluate our services. Our goal is to provide the highest quality health care possible. You are a valued customer and your opinion matters to us.

When you are done, please close the survey so that the prestamped and preprinted return mail address appears on the outside of the survey.

Thank you for helping us at the Get Well Clinic do a better job for you.

6

WRITING YOUR OWN SURVEY ITEMS

In this chapter we will discuss how to write survey questions. We will first discuss how to write quantitative questions. These are specific and global questions that ask respondents to represent their exposure to stimuli, value judgments, or reactions on a scale that is associated with numerical values.

The second part of this chapter will discuss how to write qualitative questions, or what are sometimes referred to as "open-ended questions." These are the questions that ask respondents to write comments to express their exposure to stimuli, value judgments, and reactions.

Writing Quantitative Items

Writing good survey items takes an enormous amount of training, time, patience, drafting, field and statistical testing, intelligence, and money. That is why it is best not to write your own items from scratch. There are many sources from which you can get patient satisfaction survey questions.

First, there are consulting firms, such as Press, Gainey Associates in South Bend, Indiana, and Dr. Raymond Carey of Parkside Associates in Chicago, Illinois, that have been designing patient satisfaction surveys for years. They will sell you their survey forms and help you to implement them at your own site. In addition, our own Patient Satisfaction Measurement System, run out of Ohio State University's College of Medicine, offers standard survey forms. Second, there are published surveys in the literature that can help you in writing your items. There is an excellent example in a recent supplemental issue of *Medical Care* (Meterko et al. 1990, pp. S45–S56). Third, your colleagues at other noncompeting hospitals may be willing to share their survey forms with you.

We are not suggesting that you must use someone else's boilerplates. Actually, we strongly discourage this since most hospitals have unique patient satisfaction measurement needs that they wish to meet. However, preexisting surveys offer you a much better starting place than a committee of 12 health care staff members attempting to hammer out their own 75 survey items from scratch. Even if you use or adapt someone else's survey forms, you may still wish to write many of your own questions. Here is a set of guidelines on how to do this well.

Guidelines on Writing Good Quantitative Survey Questions

Avoid leading questions

It is important not to phrase each survey question in a way that may lead the respondents into a specific answer. Survey questions like "Didn't you think the food service was excellent? SD   D   N   S   SA" may lead the respondent toward a positive response set bias. Remember, respondents often want to give socially desirable responses; that is, they want to make positive or pleasant comments about their stay or visit, more often than not. Do not further exacerbate this bias with leading questions.

    Sometimes people can get confused over what is and is not a leading question. The above example is leading because the prefacing stem, "Didn't you think," implies that respondents should agree with the statement. If the question is worded "Food services were excellent. SD   D   N   A   SA," respondents are not told whether they should or should not agree, and they have substantially more freedom of choice in how they answer.

Measure only one idea within each survey item

Survey items should measure only one feeling, response, impression, thought, value judgment, or reaction. Consider the following example: "The nurses were courteous and respectful. SD D N A SA." If the respondent circles *A*, to what is he or she agreeing? Does the respondent believe that the nurses were courteous, respectful, or both? In designing a survey, it is best to break such questions into more than one item.

Assume the respondent knows very little about
health care concepts, ideas, and language

Some patients will know more than others about health care and its terminology. If the survey is written for a knowledge level more advanced than the level most respondents possess, then the responses will be unreliable and invalid. Consider the following examples:

1. The EKG service staff was courteous.   SD D N SA A

2. The EKG service staff was courteous.
   (EKG service staff runs tests to trace
   your heartbeat.)   SD D N SA A

The second example is preferred because it defines "EKG" for the respondent. Now all respondents will be working from the same knowledge base in answering this question, which, in turn, should increase measurement reliability and validity.

Attempt to see things through the patient's eyes

When conducting survey research it is all too easy to forget whose ideas are the most important. Survey designers often fall prey to the "false consensus bias"—they think that what they perceive, feel, and believe is similar to what their respondents perceive, feel, and believe (Fiske and Taylor 1984). Research evidence in social psychology has indicated that this is simply not the case (Fiske and Taylor 1984, pp. 82–83). False consensus bias presents a substantial risk in survey design since the survey designer could lose sight of the "phenomenonology" of the health care event from the patient's perspective, as the following will explain.

A survey will be valid only to the extent that it captures aspects of the event or phenomenon you are trying to evaluate. In this case, we are trying to evaluate patients' perceptions of their hospital stay or clinic visit. For the survey to be valid, it must measure events as experienced and perceived by the patient, not the survey designer/researcher. If it is measured in terms of the researcher's perceptions, the survey may not be valid in terms of the patients' perceptions. This, naturally, defeats the purpose of patient satisfaction measurement.

Consider the following examples to better understand this point. The survey researcher, trying to determine the level of pain felt by the patient, might ask, "How much physical inconvenience did you experience after your surgery?" Patients may not equate "physical inconvenience" with "pain felt" and may thus misinterpret the question, although answering it honestly in their eyes. As a second example, consider the use of the word "responsive." To a survey researcher, "responsive" is a term that might be easily understood. To the patient, "responsive" may be better understood through the phrases "got there in a hurry," "came when I needed help," "answered all of my questions without hesitating," or "refilled my ice water frequently."

The objective, then, is to write survey items from the patient's perspective, not the researcher's perspective, to the greatest extent possible. This can be accomplished in a few ways.

1. Try to put yourself into the patient's mind.

2. Run focus groups on patient satisfaction, and listen to the words, concepts, and language of inpatients.

3. Pretest all of your survey items with actual patient populations. Ask patients how they are interpreting the items on your survey.

4. Ask patient relations staff to help you in understanding how patients perceive their health care experience.

5. Ask for help from clinical staff, who have listened to and heard patients express their opinions for years.

Be specific in how you write the content of your survey questions

Many survey questions generate unreliable data because they are written ambiguously. Consider the following two examples:

1. The food was appealing.   SD D N A SA

2. The food was presented in an
   appealing manner.   SD D N A SA

In the first example, respondents may be unclear about what aspect of appealing they are supposed to judge or react to—appealing taste, smell, or presentation? What may happen is that 30 percent of the respondents will refer to smell, 50 percent taste, and 20 percent presentation. The result is unreliable data, with which the manager can do nothing. The second example specifies exactly what aspect of appealing we are trying to measure—presentation. The result will be useful data. All survey items should be scrutinized to ensure content specificity.

Clearly define your referent persons

Many patient satisfaction questions refer to either specific providers or to groups of providers. Differentiating between these two is vital to survey research. Consider the following two items:

1. My doctor treated me with dignity.   SD D N A SA

2. My doctors treated me with dignity.   SD D N A SA

These two items can have entirely different meanings. The first may be useless unless we know to which individual doctor the patient is referring. Suppose the respondent answers *SD* to item 1 above. To whom is the respondent referring? It could be a doctor she saw in the emergency room, the medical resident on call during the night she arrived, or two medical students who stopped by to ask her how she was doing. We can never be sure what the respondent was thinking when answering the question.

Item 2, although limited, is more acceptable. Here, we are asking patients to make an aggregate assessment of all doctors with whom they came in contact. However, this item may not give us the specificity of information we desire. We may get a global impression of the respondent's view of all doctors. Or we may get the respondent's impression of a single doctor who had a dramatic impact on that patient's care, such as one physician out of six who was grossly rude. In the latter case, not all physicians would necessarily be evenly weighted in the respondent's mind.

The first item might be partially remedied by adding the clause "...in charge of my case"—for example, "The doctor who was in charge of my case treated me with dignity." If the patient knows who this doctor is, then we are making the referent person clear to the patient. Thus, theoretically, the data should only refer to the "doctor in charge." An alternative is to ask patients to write down the name of their primary physician and then have them respond to specific questions referring to that physician. Unfortunately, this approach is not foolproof. First, patients may not recall the name of their doctor. Second, patients may not remember which doctor was "in charge" of their case. Third, we may get data on only one doctor, although many may have been heavily involved in the care of a patient. Fourth, respondents may feel threatened about evaluating a single doctor. All of these factors could lead to unreliable data.

One way out of this morass, albeit not without its own problems, is to use the phrase "who was in charge of my case," and then determine who the physician was by using the encoded mailing label on the survey. Beware of this approach, however, because the encoded label may not be perfectly accurate. For instance, the physician identification number on the encoded label might refer to the admitting doctor in the intensive care unit or the emergency room and not to the doctor the patient was referring to in his or her responses. Hence, great care must be taken in interpreting patients' responses. If you are uncomfortable with the potential for error this creates, then the best you may be able to do is ask the question about all doctors (item 2). At this stage in our work we are simply not sure about which is the best way to handle this dilemma.

For those of you who are in large academic teaching hospitals, deciding which doctor is really being evaluated and whether to use "doctor" or "doctors" can be very difficult. There are the attendants, the junior and senior residents, the interns, and the medical students. At the Ohio State University Hospitals, the plural "doctors" is used, and the operating assumption is that ultimately, and as stated in medical staff bylaws, it is the attending physician who is responsible for the actions, decisions, and behaviors of all house officers or medical students reporting to him or her for a specific rotation and time period. Reporting of results are under the attending physician's name and service. Your hospital's environment may be structured differently, and you will need to consider carefully what is the most viable approach for your hospital and physicians.

A different method is to rely on open-ended questions. Following the specific quantitative items about the "physician in charge" or "physicians involved in your care," open-ended qualitative questions about physician care could be asked: "Were there other physicians with whom you came in contact whom you would like to comment on?" This question partially gets at the problem of limiting the response set to only one physician. Moreover, our data show that patients will cite specific examples of physicians as well as their positive or negative experiences with them. True, this is not the most systematic way to measure satisfaction with physicians since some patients tend to respond to open-ended items more than others. Nonetheless, qualitative comments about physicians' care may generate the most specific, valid, and useful information of all and are explored in more depth in Chapter 9.

What about nurses? Don't we face an even more difficult referent problem with this group of providers? There are more of them (compared to physicians), thus making identification more difficult. There are solutions to this problem, however. First, the researcher might ask the patient to comment on nursing care in general, for example, "Nurses were respectful." Then the patient satisfaction researcher can use the encoded label to determine the patient's nursing discharge unit. There is, however, a problem with this idea also. Many patients get transferred from floor to floor and service to service within the hospital. Hence, some patients may be referring to nurses who were not in the encoded nursing discharge unit, leading to erroneous conclusions.

We have recently tried a second approach and asked patients to rate their perception of the quality of nursing care for specific shifts:

The nursing care on the following shifts was excellent:
Weekday

Morning to afternoon	SD	D	N	A	SA
Afternoon to midnight	SD	D	N	A	SA
Midnight to early morning	SD	D	N	A	SA

Weekend

Morning to afternoon	SD	D	N	A	SA
Afternoon to midnight	SD	D	N	A	SA
Midnight to early morning	SD	D	N	A	SA

Early results seem to indicate that this will yield useful information.

Third, qualitative data again may be the most useful in terms of identifying specific nurses who did excellent work, as well as those whose interaction with, or care of, a given patient was not successful. A general, open-ended item like "Please make any additional comments on the quality of nursing care you received in the space below" will yield a plethora of general and specific information. The question "Please identify the name of any nurse who made your stay more pleasant and explain what he or she did" will yield even more specific information.

Collecting accurate information on specific providers is possible, though not without its difficulties. Combining quantitative questions that are directed at groups of providers with qualitative questions that are directed at deriving more specific information may be the best method one can use at this stage in patient satisfaction research.

Write items with a specific and clear level and unit of analysis in mind (a corollary to the above guideline)

Historically, a major problem with patient satisfaction surveys has been the lack of attention paid to specifying the level or unit of analysis. Traditionally, data were collected at the hospitalwide or clinicwide level. There was nothing wrong with this per se. However, managers might throw up their hands in despair and bemoan: "Now what? How do I know which of my medical services or nursing units are above or below the hospitalwide average? How do I know where to make problem-specific, ameliorative interventions?"

The rule in patient satisfaction measurement is to design your survey so that you can analyze your data at the smallest unit of analysis possible. For instance, having data that can be broken down by nursing discharge unit or nursing shift is far better than having only overall nursing department level data. The question is, How do we do this?

One answer you already know—the encoded labeling system described in Chapter 4. If you do not decide to use the encoded label, then patients must recall their location in the hospital, wing or building in the hospital, medical service, physician, and/or room number. Our data show that patients, for many good reasons, have tremendous difficulty remembering these items accurately (see Chapter 4 for more discussion on this point).

A second answer is to write items that incorporate language pertinent to the unit of analysis you are interested in exploring. For instance, you may wish to write items specific to your hospital's emergency department or intensive care unit.

Always ask, What will I learn from this survey question?

In putting together patient satisfaction surveys, it is all too easy to ask questions that ostensibly sound great, but offer very little useful information to the health care manager. One way to avoid this is to write out a question you are considering for inclusion and fabricate data that you might receive back in response to this question—for example, 32 percent said Strongly Agree, 21 percent said Agree, and so on. Next, assuming that these were your results, ask yourself the following questions:

- What are they telling me?
- What might they mean?
- Are they going to help me identify operational strengths or weaknesses?
- Are they going to help me solve problems?
- Will I be able to use these results?
- Will I believe these results?
- Will these results teach me something important about my patients, my staff, my hospital, and the care we render?
- Are there other items in the survey that will help me understand the results I am getting better than the survey question I am currently reviewing?

Asking and answering these questions can help you write more useful survey items.

Ask positively and negatively worded questions

Consider the following two survey items:

1. My nurses did not seem confident in
   managing my care.   SD   D   N   A   SA

2. My nurses seemed confident in
   managing my care.   SD   D   N   A   SA

The first item is negatively worded; the second is positively worded. Both kinds of items should be used in patient satisfaction survey research. The split does not have to be 50/50. We believe that inserting about one negatively worded item among every four or five positively worded items will accrue at least two benefits. First, readers are more likely to stay "on task" if they come across an item that is not presented in the expected pattern. An unexpected pattern may help to maintain the respondents' attention and reduce skimming or speed-reading through the survey. Second, and similarly, inserting negatively worded items may lower the chances of respondents getting into a response set pattern such as circling all Agrees down the survey page.

The problem you will face with negatively worded items is more political than methodological. We have found that health care managers, nurses, and doctors are threatened by them. They believe that negatively worded questions will predispose a negative response. Even when we tell our managers that the computer programs reverse (mirror) the raw scores (1 = 5, 2 = 4, 3 = 3, 4 = 2, 5 = 1) and that the data are then reported in the positive, managers and clinicians alike remain resistant.

We believe that if resistance is shown, then you should not force the issue. Once confidence in your organization's patient satisfaction measurement system is established, it should be easier to receive approval for rewording some of the positively phrased items into negatively phrased items.

Get input from others when writing items

For both political and methodological reasons it is important to ask for input from physicians, nursing, ancillary, administration, housekeeping, and dietary staff on what kind of questions they would like to have asked. Obviously, there are important political implications in terms of getting the health care team to buy into the survey process. However, there is a strong methodological payoff, too. Your staff will have more content knowledge about their clinical and nonclinical areas than the patient satisfaction researcher. Therefore, they are more likely to identify key issues and critical incidents—stimuli—in the patient's stay or clinic visit that should be included in the survey.

Measure patient perceptions of treatment quality

It is often argued that lay patients are unable to assess the quality of clinical treatment they receive. This argument is valid only if one considers the provider's perception as the only valid one. Patients, in our judgment, can assess the quality of clinical treatment, at the very least, from their perception. As long as it is understood that it is their perception, it seems critical to hear what they have to say about their clinical care.

Certainly, patients can evaluate how much comfort or discomfort they experienced. They can also assess if clinical services were delivered efficiently and without undue delay or confusion. Patients can probably evaluate even far more. Many have a comparative knowledge base to draw from due to previous health care experience. They may know that it should not take seven sticks to start an IV or that their antibiotic should not be delivered, on average, one hour off schedule. Many patients remind providers of clinical treatment factors that perhaps they should not need to be reminded of: "Hold it, I'm allergic to penicillin and the bottle you're holding says 'Pen VK 500 mg'" or "Didn't anyone tell you I'm diabetic? I can't eat this meal they gave me."

Thus, we agree with Nelson and Niederberger's (1990) implication that quality patient satisfaction measurement of the 1990s may indeed need to include patients' evaluations of the quality of clinical treatment they received.

Measure patient perception of clinical and psychological outcomes

For many of the same reasons just cited, patient evaluation of clinical and psychological outcomes should be measured. For example, patients can assess whether or not they are better off from their health care encounter. As important, they can accurately assess if their quality of life (for example, mobility, psychological status, pain) is better or worse due to their health care experience. As Nelson and Niederberger (1990) note:

> At the minimum, the research literature and this sample suggests that patient satisfaction surveys could usefully include more content relating to continuity-of-care issues, patients' expectations, and patient assessments of the *effect of the encounter on their health* (p. 422, emphasis added).

How might this be accomplished? At the most basic level, we could ask a question like "I am better off for seeking medical care at the Better Health Outpatient Clinic. SD   D   N   A   SA." Or we could get more specific—for instance, asking surgery patients, "Did you experience any unplanned complications?" or "Surgery improved the quality of my life. SD   D   N   A   SA."

It is quite clear that patient satisfaction measurement in the next decade will need to include measures of both patients' perceptions of the clinical treatment they received and the self-assessed desirability of their medical outcomes.

Measure specific behaviors and attitudes in addition to general impressions

Consider the following item: "The nurses were nice. SD D N A SA." This item measures patients' general perception of their nursing care. However, what do the patients' responses to this question tell us? For instance, if the nurses were not nice, do we know why? Was it poor listening skills, lack of empathy, roughness when moving the patient, or indifference to family questions that caused the patient to complain? Despite this caveat, these kinds of general perceptions can still be worth measuring. They can, for instance, be very helpful in assessing the type of image and climate the health care organization is projecting. For example, one PSMS contract research client wanted to assess what kind of image its outpatient clinic was projecting to consumers. These general perception questions proved very useful.

Let's turn our attention to a different kind of survey question. Please consider the following survey items:

1. The nurses carefully listened to my
   questions.   SD D N A SA

2. The nurses responded to my call
   button requests quickly.   SD D N A SA

3. The nurses who worked with me were
   rude.   SD D N A SA

These offer a different type of advantage. They ask respondents to comment on specific behaviors or attitudes among the nursing staff. The data generated will allow nursing management to determine if behaviors and attitudes deemed desirable are occurring. Moreover, if they are not occurring, the nature of the item tells the health care manager exactly what behaviors and attitudes the patients feel are lacking. Suppose 43 percent of the respondents Agree or Strongly Agree that the nursing staff was rude. This tells nursing management exactly how their nurses need to improve. What is more, if the encoded label is used, this "rudeness problem" can be analyzed and broken down by nursing discharge unit, adding to the specificity of the analysis. When the analysis is completed, nursing management can then ask the next logical and crucial questions: Why are nurses in 3N, 4N, and 2S being perceived as rude more often than nurses in other units? Is it their behavior? Or is it due to the acuity and age of the patients?

Including items that look at the behavior and attitude of your staff is critical to effective patient satisfaction measurement. It becomes particularly important in reinforcing desirable behaviors and in changing less desirable behaviors.

Take your time developing patient satisfaction survey items

It is a mistake to rush through a few drafts of a survey and then go to press. Writing good survey items takes an enormous amount of time. It is not uncommon to go through eleven or twelve thorough revisions before reaching a final draft. It is amazing how survey items can seem perfectly wonderful one day, and then the next day glaring and fatal flaws will be quickly identified.

The following is a classic example of this kind of mistake. Under time pressure, we wrote a survey item that asked, "Would you recommend Health Hospital to family and friends?" We agonized over the dual focus of this question (to family and friends) and decided to include it in this particular instance. We printed and distributed our survey with this item and collected a great deal of good, usable information. However, since we were rushing and focusing only on the dual focus flaw, we missed a second key point. We did not attempt to measure the patient's "behavioral intent" (Fishbein and Ajzen 1975) to return to the hospital. We could have assessed this through a question such as "Would you return to Health Hospital if you needed medical care in the future?" An assessment of your patient's behavioral intent to return is perhaps as important, if not more important, than evaluating whether the patient will recommend your hospital.

The ground rules are simple here:

- Take your time putting your survey together.
- Have doctors give input into doctor items, nurses give input into nursing items, and so on.
- Have doctors give input into nursing items, nurses give input into doctor items, and so on.
- Review your survey questions numerous times before using them.
- Ask yourself the questions listed previously in this chapter about what each survey item will be able to tell you.
- Pretest your questions with consumers before finalizing your survey. Ask consumers to comment on how well they understood the questions in the survey and how they interpreted them.
- Have your health care organization's attorney review your items to make sure that there are not potential legal problems with your survey questions and format.

Use response scales intelligently

In quantitative methods, response scales can be as important as the survey items themselves. Aside from some of the more obvious suggestions, such as keeping the scales simple and easy to understand, here are some additional ideas that may help.

Use continuous scales whenever possible. Continuous scales ask respondents to select a value on some alphanumeric continuum that best expresses how they feel. Examples are shown in Exhibit 6.1.

Exhibit 6.1 Examples of Continuous Scales

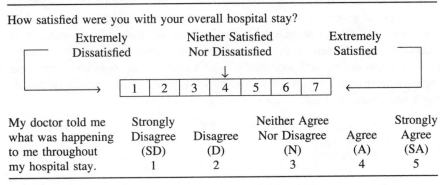

There are some important assumptions and suggestions about continuous scales that need to be made, understood, and implemented. First, the interval distance between units on the scale must be the same. For instance, in the seven-point satisfaction scale in Exhibit 6.1, the distance between choices 2 and 3 represents the same amount of satisfaction as the distance between choices 5 and 6.

Second, the scale should be in a constant ascending or descending direction; for example, always place Extremely Dissatisfied as the leftmost point on the scale and Extremely Satisfied as the rightmost point on the scale. Third, the scale must be anchored: There must be descriptive words corresponding to various points on the alphanumeric scale; for example, in Exhibit 6.1, a *1* is equivalent to the phrase Strongly Disagree and a *5* is equivalent to the phrase Strongly Agree. Not all parts of the scale need to be anchored, but anchors should occur at equal intervals on the scale. At the very minimum we recommend anchoring the lowest point, the midpoint(s), and the highest point on the scale.

Except in cases where you have no choice, avoid Yes/No dichotomous scales. In fact, if possible, also avoid trichotomous scales, such as Yes/Maybe/No. There are a few reasons for this. The most important is maximizing the opportunity for generating variance (offering respondents a relatively wide range of choices) in the patient's response set. Yes/No questions have only two choices, which may constrain the respondent from expressing partial or ambivalent judgments. The respondent may have liked 80 percent of the nursing service's care but, with only two choices available, may have to indicate an all-or-nothing level of satisfaction.

Use five- or seven-point continuous interval scales. Using a small number of intervals may constrain variance in response sets. Asking a Yes/No item ("Were you satisfied with your medical care?") limits the possible responses patients could give. All the gradations and degrees of satisfaction are lost if only two intervals are provided. On the other hand, using a larger number of intervals, such as a ten- or even a hundred-point scale, forces respondents to make minute differential judgments, which may not be possible. Thus, we recommend five- or seven-point continuous interval scales, although this is not a fixed rule. The following scales are examples:

	Poor	Fair	Average	Good	Excellent
1. The nursing care was	1	2	3	4	5
2. The nurses told me what was happening to me at all times	SD 1	D 2	N 3	A 4	SA 5
3. My doctor treated me gently when (s)he examined me	SD 1	D 2	N 3	A 4	SA 5

Include midpoints on your scale. Although some survey researchers use response scales that omit the midpoint on a continuous interval scale, we strongly discourage this practice. The midpoint is omitted in the following example:

	SD	D	A	SA
I experienced more pain in the hospital than I should have	1	2	3	4

The argument is that this will force respondents to express a positive or negative value judgment or reaction in response to a given stimulus. Without a midpoint, respondents are structurally excluded from sitting on the fence and offering an in-between response. In effect, these kinds of scales become forced judgment scales for respondents who may feel ambivalent.

We encourage patient satisfaction researchers to avoid no-midpoint scales. Midpoints allow people to demonstrate if they feel neutral about particular issues. Hospital experiences can be average, and people do feel ambivalent—comme ci, comme ça. How many times have you heard patients say, "The food was neither good nor bad. Sort of in-between." To omit midpoints is to impose a distribution of responses on patients that may not truly reflect how they feel and results in less measurement validity because we are no longer measuring the true level of judgment or reaction our patients may wish to express.

Additionally, excluding the midpoint violates the assumption cited earlier that the unit distance between all intervals in the scale must be the same. The conceptual and operational difference (distance) between Strongly Disagree and Disagree is not the same as the conceptual and operational difference between Disagree and Agree when the midpoint (Neither Agree Nor Disagree) is omitted. If this assumption is violated, the use of more powerful statistics (statistics that are more likely to be sensitive to true differences) will be less valid.

Do not insult your respondents

With the diversity of most patient populations, it is all to easy to offend someone with your survey. For instance, writing items that refer to doctors in the masculine is both sexist and inaccurate. Or consider the following item: "Only poor people come to this hospital for care. SD   D   N   A   SA." This item may be offensive to many of your patients, both poor and wealthy.

The message to the survey designer is simple: Aside from thoroughly evaluating all of your items before going into the field with them, review the appropriateness of your items from ethical, religious, socioeconomic, gender, race, and marital perspectives.

Market research

As noted in Chapter 1, you can write quantitative items for market research purposes:

Out of the following factors, please select the two most important ones that made you choose our outpatient clinic for your medical needs:

___ physician referral   ___ reputation of clinic

___ network physician   ___ availability of specific

___ short waiting times   specialist

___ location of clinic   ___ lower out-of-pocket costs
near home
___ family member or friend
___ on-site pharmacy   referral

___ on-site child care   ___ ease of parking

The main caution here is not to confound the purposes of your survey with the methods. Specifically, you do not want the "marketing" items to contaminate the reliability and validity of the patient satisfaction data you are trying to collect.

Be careful of using rank order or forced-choice questions

Questions that ask respondents to rank their value judgments and reactions can generate deceiving data and erroneous conclusions. Consider the following example:

Please rank the following groups of people in terms of the quality of care you received from them. Place a 1 next to the group you felt delivered the best care, a 2 next to the group that delivered the second-best level of care, and so on. No ties, please.

Sample of a Completed Survey

Provider Group	Rank 1 to 4
Nurses	4
Doctors	3
X-ray	1
Laboratory	2

The basic problem with this approach is that we have no idea just how much better x-ray staff are than the laboratory staff group ranked just below them. For example, the former could rate an "excellent plus" in the respondent's mind, and the latter could rate an "excellent." The rank values of 1 through 4 are unanchored, making it difficult to determine what these values truly mean. Hence, rank ordering may create differences that are artificial, and even meaningless. From the above example, nurses, who ranked last, may be in this patient's mind "excellent minus."

The same problem can occur with what are referred to as "forced-choice" methodologies. Consider the following example:

1. Nurses delivered better care than the
   doctors. _____ Yes _____ No

2. Nurses delivered better care than
   laboratory staff. _____ Yes _____ No

3. Doctors delivered better care than
   laboratory staff. _____ Yes _____ No

In effect, forced-choice questions like these can impose variations in value judgments and reactions that may not truly reflect the patient's value judgments and reactions.

Measure value judgments and reactions to both the frequency of stimuli and the intensity of stimuli

Some stimuli need to be measured along two dimensions: (1) how often the stimulus occurs, and (2) the intensity with which the stimulus is experienced. Perhaps the best examples can be found in nursing and physician care items:

(*Frequency*) I was very satisfied with the number of times I saw my doctor during my hospital stay. SD D N A SA

(*Intensity*) I was very satisfied with how much time the doctor spent with me when he/she visited. SD D N A SA

Sometimes it makes sense to just measure the presence or absence of certain stimuli

In the PSMS, we have determined that it can often be useful to measure the stimulus without tying it to a value judgment or reaction in the same question. For example, you might ask outpatients:

When did the doctor arrive for your appointment:

_____ Early

_____ On time

_____ Late

These results can be used later to help you analyze your data in more depth. In the above example, you could analyze overall satisfaction with physician care and break it down by each of the above three groups. Here, one might hypothesize that the "early" or "on time" group will be associated with higher physician satisfaction ratings than the group of respondents who check "late."

Seeing What You've Learned

Below are 12 survey items. Can you determine what is wrong with each of them?

1. The nurses were kind and helpful. SD D N A SA (*Answer*: Two concepts are being measured within one question.)

2. The dietary staff was pleasant. SD D N A SA (*Answer*: No midpoint on response scales.)

3. I received my meds on time. SD D N A SA (*Answer*: "Meds" is lingo—language the patient may not understand.)

4. The doctors were great. SD D N A SA (*Answer*: As a general impression item this is fine. However, nothing about the physicians' specific behaviors or attitudes are being measured.)

5. Didn't you think the food was better than you thought it would be? SD D N A SA (*Answer*: Leading question.)

6. The food was served hot. SD D N A SA (*Answer*: Type is too small.)

7. Door knobs and handles in the patient rooms were easy to find. SD D N A SA (*Answer*: You probably would have no use for the information you would collect from this item.)

8. In light of your last two hospital stays and given that you are over 40 years of age, how satisfied were you with the kind of nonclinical treatment you received from the billing staff at the time of your discharge following your hospitalization? (If you had less than two hospital stays over the last year and are 40 years of age or younger, please move on to the next question.) [Response scale] (*Answer*: Too convoluted. Too many conditions for the respondent to follow.)

9. How was the care you received from them? [Response scale] (*Answer*: Referent is not clearly delineated in this example—who are "them?")

10. The nursing gals were great. SD D N A SA (*Answer*: Sexist, and also inaccurate since the number of male nurses has increased over the last two decades.)

11. The nurses did not respond to my calls fast enough. SD   D   N   A   SA (*Answer*: Nothing is wrong with this item. Some negatively worded items are encouraged.)

12. The nursing care was better than the medical care I received from my physician(s). SD   D   N   A   SA (*Answer*: This is a forced-choice item that could generate artificial differences between the two groups.)

Writing Qualitative or Open-Ended Survey Questions

As discussed earlier, qualitative or open-ended survey questions are designed to give patients an opportunity to express their value judgments and reactions to their health care experience in words. Also, as noted in previous chapters, qualitative measurement is probably greatly underused in patient satisfaction measurement. This is unfortunate since we have found that often qualitative data offer the most useful information for health care managers.

What follows are some guidelines on writing qualitative questions. Again, these are guidelines only and are not fixed and rigid rules.

Guidelines for Writing Qualitative Items

Guidelines for writing quantitative items also apply here

Many of the suggestions above apply to the development of qualitative survey items. It goes without saying that simplicity and clarity are crucial. Also, make your referent clear within the qualitative items so that respondents know what or whom they are expressing value judgments and reactions about. And, as is always the case, think through what types of information the qualitative items will generate. Speaking with other patient satisfaction researchers to see what kinds of items worked well for them will help you write more successful qualitative items.

Include qualitative items within major survey sections

As noted earlier, include qualitative items within each major section of your survey. For example, you may want to include the following two qualitative items after both the physician and nursing sections of your survey:

1. Additional comments about doctors
2. Additional comments about the nursing care you received

Include a general comment item on your survey

Because patient satisfaction surveys cannot capture the totality of every respondent's health care experience, it is sensible to close your survey with a general comment item, such as this:

> Are there other aspects about your care and the services you received that you wish to comment on?

You even might consider being very nonspecific in how you write your last general item (for example, by just asking for "general comments").

It can be useful to focus the respondent's qualitative comments

Although items like "General Comments" and "Other Comments" are helpful, it is also useful to focus the respondent on more specific issues. The above-mentioned examples of the physician and nursing items are consistent with this goal. However, you can go further. For instance, you might ask the respondent the following:

> Please list one or two recommendations that could help us at Health Hospital deliver better services and care to you.

The focus does not have to be solely negative. For example, you also might ask the respondent:

> Please comment on those aspects of your outpatient visit that you liked best.

Naturally, the above item could be made even more specific if you included a nursing, dietary, or physician referent.

Identifying individual health care staff

We recommend that when the qualitative item directs the respondent to make negative value judgments or reactions (for example, "What could we do to improve ... ?"), the referent should never be a single person, but instead a group of persons. For instance, we would not recommend your asking:

> Please identify any nurse or physician, by name and location, who might have done a better job in delivering medical care and services to you.

There are a variety of reasons why this should not be done. First, it would be far too threatening to your health care staff, and it would undermine their confidence and trust in the system. Second, the survey system might be perceived as primarily negative by your health care staff—a "witch-hunting device." Remember, an important philosophical perspective to effective patient satisfaction measurement is to keep it positive. Third, you do not need to ask these questions, because patients typically provide the names of health care staff who they feel have done a less than meritorious job anyway.

What you can do, however, is ask for generic negative feedback, such as "How can we improve our housekeeping services?" This will appear less threatening to health care staff as long as there are questions concerning all departments and no one group (for example, housekeeping) is singled out.

Although we strongly discourage you from asking respondents to identify poor performers through specific qualitative items, we encourage you to identify individual staff who did their jobs particularly well. The following are two examples of such items:

> Was there anyone who helped make your outpatient visit more pleasant (name, clinic location, job title)?

> Were there any physicians who you felt went above and beyond the call of duty (name and location)?

Identify underlying reasons and motivations

Use qualitative items to identify the *why* behind the *what*. Qualitative items can be an excellent way to identify the underlying reasons behind respondents giving certain value judgments and reactions. Consider the following as an example of how this can be accomplished through qualitative items:

> If you would return to the Better Health Clinic for your future health care needs, why would you make our clinic your choice again?

> If you would not want to return to Better Health Clinic for your future health care needs, why would you choose to go to another clinic?

Market research and qualitative items

Consider the following examples to help you get a better idea of how qualitative items can be helpful in market research.

> Please identify any new medical service you would like our outpatient clinic to offer.

> Please list the main reasons why you use our outpatient clinic.

These, and many other open-ended questions like them, can be designed with the marketing department's help and input.

Be balanced

Qualitative items can lead respondents to focus on the positive or negative aspects of their health care experience. However, this does not mean you should focus only on one and not the other. When you write your qualitative items, review them to ensure that you are not asking respondents to focus too much on the positive or negative.

Conclusion

This chapter has explored many of the issues pertinent to writing effective patient satisfaction survey research questions. Our closing words to you are to be aware of all the unexpected and possible contingencies that can arise from writing survey questions. Hard and diligent development work—iterations, drafting, discussing, multiple input—is good preventive medicine, but it is never perfect. The bad news is that after the fact, you will always think that you could have done a better job. The good news is that as time goes on, your survey should get better and better.

7

SURVEY DISTRIBUTION, RESPONSE RATES, AND SAMPLING

Should you distribute surveys to every discharged patient, or should you sample patients periodically? Should you hand the surveys out at the time of discharge or distribute them through the mail after discharge? How do we know if we have a generalizable set of survey responses? Do we need to survey nonrespondents? These and similar questions will be addressed in this chapter.

How Often and How Many Discharged Patients Should We Sample?

Like so many questions pertaining to patient satisfaction survey research, the ostensible answer to this question is easy, while the more thoughtful one is complex. Following are some guidelines that will help you in deciding on the frequency and intensity of your sampling procedure.

What Are Your Objectives?

The goals of your patient satisfaction measurement system will have an important bearing on this issue. Suppose your hospital is very committed to developing a one-to-one relationship with each of its customers. Under these circumstances, surveying all of your discharges may make sense. The same might be true if your hospital considers the patient satisfaction survey as an important marketing and community image-building tool. If this is not an objective, then sampling on, say, a quarterly basis may be sufficient. Assess what you wish to accomplish through your system and let that guide you in your sampling decisions.

What Can You Afford?

Cost is always a mitigating factor. Not all hospitals or outpatient clinics can afford to survey all discharges. The mailing costs assumed in surveying 12,000 discharges per year will be substantially higher than the costs of surveying only a quarter of this population. However, some health care managers may get confused on this issue. Although it obviously costs more to process 12,000 surveys, the variable costs are not that large compared to the fixed costs—that is, the cost of processing 12,000 surveys will not equal four times the cost of processing 3,000 surveys. In fact, it will amount to somewhat less. It is the generation of detailed feedback reports and complex data analysis that can be so costly.

Our recommendation is to survey as many of your discharges as you can afford. The reason has relatively less to do with getting a representative sample and more to do with marketing, effectively communicating with your community, risk management, and performance accountability.

If you are unable to survey all discharges, then consider four survey periods per year—quarterly sampling—evenly spread out over the course of the year. (Establishing six survey periods is another alternative.) These four survey periods should be between six and eight weeks long. All discharges will be sent surveys during this period of time, although this will depend on the total number of discharges or outpatient visits in a given year. The crucial component in quarterly sampling is generating a "critical mass" of respondents: We wish to survey enough people so that our breakdown analyses by nursing discharge unit, by medical service, by admitting physician, and so forth have sufficient numbers of respondents to meaningfully interpret the data at these smaller levels of analysis.

Consider the following example to help clarify this point. Suppose you have 10,000 discharges per year and you conduct four 4-week samplings. This means that about 3,000+ surveys [10,000 × (4 × 4)/52] will be distributed. Also, suppose you get about a 30 percent response rate; that is, 900 surveys are returned for the entire year, or about 225 surveys are returned per quarter. If you have six major nursing units, then there will be roughly 38 returned surveys that can be correlated back to each of those units each quarter. And herein lies the rub!

Even if you can say that the 225 respondents are a representative sample of your total population of discharges, your nursing staff (in this example) may feel uncomfortable being evaluated on just 38 discharges per unit for that quarter. The world's most renowned statistician can tell these nurses that this is a valid sample, but the nurses may not believe these data because they are still based on only 38 cases. This has more to do with the psychological responses to sampling and less to do with the mathematical science of sampling. If your nurses simply cannot buy into the idea that 38 is a significant critical mass, then the patient satisfaction measurement tool has lost a great deal of its efficacy.

The problem is not just at the nursing discharge unit level of analysis. CEOs too may be psychologically uncomfortable reporting quarterly patient satisfaction results to their board. They too may simply not be able to conceptually accept the idea that the impressions of 225 respondents is equivalent to the impressions of 3,000+ total discharges for a given quarter. What's more, will the hospital or clinic board and medical staff executive committee believe this? To make sample size matters worse, you may have a 30 percent response rate, but 5 percent of the returned data may contain a great deal of missing data. This makes the reportable sample sizes even smaller.

It is not that health care professionals are lousy statisticians. The issue is largely psychological. When one's job performance is being evaluated, which is a mega issue to most health care employees, small though representative samples may not be acceptable. The idea is to build up your sample size to as large a number as is both possible and practical: If you go to a quarterly system, survey for more than four- or five-week intervals each quarter. This translates into the time frame for a 48- to 52-week year shown in Figure 7.1. The quarterly sampling time system displayed in Figure 7.1 is a guideline only. Smaller hospitals will probably need to survey for longer periods of time to build up a sufficient psychological and mathematical

Figure 7.1   Timing on Quarterly Survey Sampling System

Quarter 1	$\longrightarrow$	Survey for 8 consecutive weeks No surveying for 5 consecutive weeks
Quarter 2	$\longrightarrow$	Survey for 8 consecutive weeks No surveying for 5 consecutive weeks
Quarter 3	$\longrightarrow$	Survey for 8 consecutive weeks No surveying for 5 consecutive weeks
Quarter 4	$\longrightarrow$	Survey for 8 consecutive weeks No surveying for 5 consecutive weeks

critical mass of surveys. Moreover, response rates may also influence how many discharges you sample.

What about biannual survey systems? Two survey periods of 16 weeks in length will, theoretically, net the same number of respondents as four 8-week survey periods. However, if the survey periods are shortened, the critical mass problem (psychologically and mathematically) could present itself.

We do not wish to ignore the important relationship between sample size and the plus or minus error that is associated with patient satisfaction scores. This is especially true as units of analysis get smaller. If sample sizes get too small, then the plus or minus error rates associated with each score may be unacceptable to the patient satisfaction researcher and manager. Before any sampling decisions are made, consult with a trained statistician who can explain the relationship between error and sample size.

How Should Surveys Be Distributed?

Although we suggest mailing the surveys to patients shortly after they are discharged, there are many options for distribution to consider, each having its own strengths and weaknesses.

Choice 1: Distributing Surveys during the Patient's Stay

Although we have read accounts where a version of this approach has been successful, we do not believe that distribution during the patient's stay is the best method for distributing surveys. The problems include the patient's uncertain levels of acuity, alertness, and motivation to complete the survey. Many patients, for instance, are medicated during their stay, which can make their survey responses less than reliable (to say the least!). The same can be said for patients who are in pain or emotionally distraught.

There is, perhaps, another problem with this approach—the totality of the inpatient stay has yet to be fully experienced and assimilated by the respondent. A patient, for example, could complete sections of the survey (for example, on nursing care) without having experienced subsequent nursing care stimuli, such as care after surgery. The situation is analogous to a restaurant's management asking its patrons to complete a questionnaire after their drinks have been served.

Another problem with this approach is that it could heighten patients' sense of vulnerability that an ancillary service or clinical provider will retaliate—during their current stay—if they evaluate his or her services and care critically, adding to what is already a positive response bias or leniency effect with many patient satisfaction surveys.

It is true that some hospital and health care incidents could be surveyed right after the time the patient experiences them. Inpatient registration and admitting are examples of this. Immediate surveying is very appealing because patients' memories should be excellent if they are surveyed right after the stimulus is experienced. However, gathering some data during the stay and then more data after the stay seems operationally difficult and costly to implement.

Choice 2: Distributing Surveys at Time of Discharge

Although others may have had successful experiences with on-site hand-distribution at discharge, the PSMS has not succeeded with this approach in outpatient settings. We see at least four problems with on-site hand-delivered surveys at the time of discharge:

1. At discharge, the inpatient leaves with flowers, plants, written medical instructions, medications, suitcases, and shopping bags. It is a cluttered and confused time. It is all too easy for the survey to get lost in the shuffle.

2. Patients at discharge may not yet feel 100 percent well. Giving them a survey at discharge may lead them to complete the survey at a time they are not in the best condition to do so. Moreover, they may be more likely to discard the survey at this time than a few days later, when they may feel healthier and better able to respond.

3. We have generally found health care staff nonsupportive in distributing surveys. Although they clearly state that they wish to comply, their behavior, in our experience, is not consistent with their intentions. In outpatient settings in which we have worked, fewer than 30 percent (estimated) of the surveys that are supposed to be hand-distributed by staff actually are handed out. Perhaps some health care staff may feel that they are contributing to career suicide—handing consumers the axe that will chop off their professional heads. Moreover, it's "just one more thing" health care staff are being asked to comply with during a day that is already filled with a "million and one other things to do." Already, there is grousing about excessive paperwork throughout American hospitals and outpatient clinics. Being asked to distribute the survey just adds fuel to the fire.

4. Related to number 3 above, this distribution process cannot be systematically controlled. Some staff will distribute surveys more conscientiously than others. The result could be a nonrepresentative sample of distributed surveys and, ultimately, respondents.

This is not to say that there are not circumstances where direct hand-distribution at discharge makes sense. When money is tight, there may be no other way. Or perhaps the hospital's or clinic's management information system is unable to generate mailing labels soon enough after discharge. If this is the case, staff who will hand-distribute surveys must receive extensive training in how to accomplish this systematically. The distribution system must be standardized. It is important that staff see and experience the benefits of distributing the survey. Otherwise, resistance is more likely to occur. In outpatient clinics we have had some recent success with hiring special staff to hand out surveys as patients leave the building. This approach is *not* recommended, however, for inpatient settings.

Choice 3: Mailing Surveys after the Inpatient Stay or Clinic Visit

Mailing surveys after the inpatient stay or clinic visit, although not perfect, seems to have a number of advantages. First, it gives the patient satisfaction researcher time to acquire information from patients' medical records and encode it on to their surveys.

Second, it allows patients to physically and psychologically assimilate their total inpatient experience. If they receive the survey four to ten days after discharge, they have had an opportunity to process the complete experience.

Third, it allows patients to complete the survey when they are less likely to be experiencing negative and potentially confounding physiological or psychological effects of their illness.

Fourth, mailed surveys give patients safer "psychological distance" from the hospital. Patients can complete the survey off site, in private, and with more assurance that they will not suffer negative consequences for their critical comments.

Of course, there are costs to this approach, both fiscal and methodological. Obviously, mailing surveys costs more. We estimate that with stuffing, labeling, sorting, and postage, the cost can run as high as $0.49 per survey, or even more. If 10,000 discharges are surveyed annually, this adds about $5,000 to your survey costs. A second problem may lie in sending the surveys to patients too long after they have left the hospital. This issue is addressed in depth in the next section.

In summary, we recommend a mailed survey approach because there is a greater chance, we believe, of generating more reliable and valid data. In addition, the response rate may increase as well. Although the costs are certainly not trivial, they pale in comparison to the costs associated with adding bias to your results and lowering your response rate.

When Should Surveys Be Mailed?

In a perfect patient satisfaction measurement system, patients would receive an encoded survey on the third to sixth day after their discharge. Generally at this time, the experience should be sufficiently assimilated, memory should still be relatively good, pain and discomfort should be somewhat allayed, the patient should feel safer, and the motivation to respond should be acceptable.

Unfortunately, it is difficult to accomplish delivery of surveys within this time frame. There are at least two limitations with which we must cope if we choose to mail surveys with encoded labels. First, the medical record is not always immediately updated at the time of discharge. Hence, to generate an encoded label with no missing data, we may need to wait three to seven days postdischarge to mail the survey with a complete encoded label. Although labels could be generated and mailings conducted on a daily basis, this can be inefficient and expensive. Hence, one typically is limited to one, or maybe two, label generation computer runs and one mailing per week. Second, the postal service will take a few days to deliver the survey.

With these limitations in mind, the PSMS project has found the following system to work reasonably well. We begin with the hope that we have about a four- to fourteen-day window in which to deliver an encoded patient satisfaction survey into the discharged patient's hands. We are not thrilled with delivery dates that exceed nine days after discharge; however, there is not much we can do unless we spend more money and generate labels and mail surveys more frequently. A schedule for mailed survey distribution might look as shown in Figure 7.2.

Close readers will note that this system presents a potential methodological confound. Specifically, not all patients are receiving surveys at the exact same time after discharge. Therefore, patients receiving the survey four days postdischarge may systematically respond differently (perhaps in more detail because their memory is keener, or more unreliably because they are still on medication) than those receiving the survey, say, more than ten days post-discharge. It is difficult for the patient satisfaction researcher to assess if this confound is creating a sampling or response bias because patients do not necessarily complete the survey the day they receive it. Some wait a week, others three days, and still others two weeks or even more. Hence, the date of survey distribution may have little bearing on the postdischarge date the respondent completes the survey.

Currently, a study is badly needed to assess if unequal time-based sampling methods, such as the one proposed above, tend to bias the data obtained from the patient satisfaction survey. This study could be done by

Figure 7.2 Sample Schedule for Mailed Survey Distribution*

> Boxed numbers indicate label
> generation and mailing dates.

August 1994

Monday	Tuesday	Wednesday	Thursday	Friday	Saturday	Sunday
1	2	3	4	[5	6	7]

Patients are discharged; no labels are
run; no surveys are sent.

Monday	Tuesday	Wednesday	Thursday	Friday	Saturday	Sunday
8	9	10	11	[12	13	14]

Generate labels for all discharges from
the previous week. Mail surveys on the
same day.

| 15 | 16 | 17 | 18 | [19 | 20 | 21] |

Generate labels for all discharges from
the previous week, and labels for
discharges August 4/5 to August 7.

| 22 | 23 | 24 | 25 | [26 | 27 | 28] |

Generate labels for all discharges from
the previous week, and labels for
discharges August 11/12 to August 14.

September

| 29 | 30 | 31 | 1 | [2 | 3 | 4] |

Generate labels for all discharges from
the previous week, and labels for
discharges August 18/19 to August 21.

*Note that in general we recommend that sampling periods not be less than six weeks. Hence, in reality, this schedule would be extended three to four more weeks than is shown in this example.

tracking the date the surveys are distributed and then asking respondents to answer the following question, "On what date did you complete this survey?" Some work in this area has been done by Meterko et al. (1990, p. S38). They find that surveys administered closer to the time of discharge yield slightly higher satisfaction ratings on three of their satisfaction scales, though they suggest that the magnitude of this effect is "of no practical importance." These researchers go on to note:

> Mode of administration [telephone vs. mail] had no effect on the factor structure [of their satisfaction scales]. Some small differences were observed between groups differing in time interval after discharge. Regardless of mode of administration, there was a smaller general factor among those surveyed later. These results must be interpreted with caution, however, due to the small sample sizes (pp. S38–S39).

Should We Use Incentives to Increase Response Rates?

As discussed in Chapter 5, providing respondents with incentives or gimmicks is not recommended to increase the response rates for a patient satisfaction survey.

Suppose you are concerned about receiving a low response rate. To prevent this, you decide to enclose a dollar bill in each survey—Better Health Clinic's personal way of saying, "A big thanks in advance." Or suppose you tell potential respondents that if they return the survey, they become eligible for a trip for two to

> Fabulous Inner-City Atlantic City. That's right. Four days and three nights at the magnificent Inner-City Motel. Go to the casinos, have delicious meals (not included), take in fabulous entertainment (not included), swim at the Taj Mahal Hotel (not included), rent a car (not included), and discover the beautiful Jersey shore and gamble your hearts out (encouraged).

The result may be that respondents will answer the survey quickly and without much thought and return it just to qualify for the "fabulous" Atlantic City trip. Some respondents may not even read the items and randomly go through the survey checking boxes and circling numbers. All this leads to substantial measurement error creeping into your measurement system.

What can also happen is that your health care organization may look foolish and unprofessional, undermining some of the marketing objectives you may wish to attain through the survey.

Finally, with some incentives (for example, the dollar bill) respondents may complete the survey out of guilt. This is not the type of underlying motivation for responding that is likely to lead to good survey data.

Should We Use Follow-Up Letters
to Increase Response Rates?

In the vast majority of survey situations, follow-up letters to nonrespondents are desirable. The problem in implementing this is that the follow-up letter could arrive 21 + days after discharge at the very earliest. By this time, some patients may have difficulty accurately recalling many detailed aspects of their stay. Moreover, follow-up letters require additional cost. If a second survey is attached to the follow-up letter, then the costs will increase even more. Also, the chances of a single respondent mistakenly completing two surveys exists.

What Can We Do to Improve Response Rates?

A few ideas on improving response rates were discussed in Chapter 5. These and some new ones will be summarized below:

1. Make your survey user-friendly. Respondents should never have to give much thought to how they should complete the scales or fill out any portion of the form.

2. Keep the survey as short as possible. As noted earlier we may have no more than ten minutes of the respondent's time.

3. Use compelling but honest language to encourage patients to participate: "Only you, our patient, can tell us just how well we did and where we need to improve our medical care and services."

4. Lay out the survey in a visually appealing manner. It should be appealing to the eye, easy to read, and should contain large type for older patients.

5. Protect or guarantee confidentiality and anonymity.

6. Tell patients that their surveys will be read.

7. Tell patients that if they have any questions they can contact someone at the hospital or outpatient clinic.

8. Get the survey into the discharged patient's hands three to ten days after discharge, if possible.

9. Pay for return mail.

10. Offer to distribute a summary of the results annually (for example, a patient satisfaction newsletter for all respondents and nonrespondents, too).

How Important Is Studying Nonrespondents?

The validity of your patient satisfaction measurement system will largely depend on the extent to which those patients who respond to your survey are demographically, clinically, and attitudinally (in terms of their patient satisfaction perceptions) equivalent to your nonrespondents. The issue here is one of "external validity" (Campbell and Stanley 1963), that is, the extent to which the results of your survey can be generalized to the total population of patients your health care organization serves.

If your respondent group is not at all similar in demographic and clinical characteristics to your nonrespondent group, then chances increase that you will not have a representative sample of respondents. This could create serious problems. Specifically, the health care manager might implement a set of costly solutions to address problems that the respondent group has identified. Although they may solve the problems addressed by your respondent group, they may be ineffectual or even harmful for the nonrespondent group.

The question we now face is, How do we know if we have a representative sample? Here are some guidelines to help you in doing this.

Analyze Your Response Sample in Depth

First, assess the demographic profile of your respondents, particularly their age, sex, and education (if available). Other information such as payer source, race, marital status, and total charges may generate useful information as well.

Second, assess the clinical profile of your respondents, including their DRGs, medical diagnostic categories, the medical services they were discharged from, acuity levels, length of stay, ICD-9 codes, and previous hospitalizations over the last 12 months.

Third, conduct a detailed analysis of how your respondent subgroups answered each survey item, calculating means, medians, standard deviation, range, and kurtosis (measure of skewness in the distribution).

The sum total of the above will give you a relatively complete profile of your response sample.

Gather Data on Your Nonrespondents

In the world of Candyland and fairy tales, we would have the same data on nonrespondents. By definition, we do not.

However, we do have some information about our nonrespondents that we may not have initially realized. Specifically, the information contained in the encoded label allows us to determine a great deal about our nonrespondent group, including their age, sex, race, DRG, medical service, ICD-9 codes, nursing discharge unit, and length of stay.

In addition, we have the nonrespondent's medical record number, and even more detailed information can be collected if we are willing to spend the money and do the work. If the respondent and nonrespondent groups possess similar demographic and clinical profiles, then that's good. Sometimes this is as good as we can get. Unfortunately, it's not good enough.

We also need to know how the nonrespondents would answer the exact same survey items—we need to know how satisfied this group was with the medical care and services they received (their patient satisfaction value judgments and reactions).

Is going this extra step overkill? We think not. Even if the demographic and clinical profiles of respondents and nonrespondents are similar, this does not mean that the nonrespondent group would have answered the survey questions similarly to the responding group. However, if both groups are demographically and clinically similar, the likelihood probably does increase that similar patient satisfaction value judgments and reactions would emerge. But it does not guarantee this.

To assess the actual situation, we must conduct patient satisfaction measurement with our nonrespondent group. As the saying goes, this is "easier said than done," since nonrespondents have already told us: "Leave me alone; I choose not to respond." We arrive at a fork in the road. We recommend taking the second fork, not the first.

Fork 1: Conduct a Mailed Patient Satisfaction Survey for Nonrespondents Only

In essence, Fork 1 involves sending out a second wave of surveys to nonrespondents only and hoping (praying if you prefer) that they will comply. Unfortunately, this too has its problems. First, the time lag between discharge and completing the nonrespondent survey could now be unacceptably long. Second, who is to say that the nonrespondents will respond to a second request after already rejecting the first? Past behavior proves, time and time again, to predict future behavior. Third, who is to say you will get a large enough sample of nonrespondents to draw meaningful conclusions? And finally, who is to say that the nonrespondents who do respond are, in fact, similar to all other nonrespondents who decline the second survey attempt in terms of their demographics, clinical dimensions, and patient satisfaction value judgments and reactions?

Fork 2: Conduct a Random Sample Telephone
Survey of Nonrespondents

A random sample telephone survey has a better chance of working because we can sample with replacement; when a nonrespondent says, "Leave me alone you creep. I'm meditating," and hangs up the phone, you can let the Ping-Pong balls roll and randomly select another nonrespondent. This method is not perfect either, for the same reason given above—the repeat nonresponders (those who declined twice) may not be similar to the nonrespondents who did respond to the telephone survey. What's more, you are now comparing survey responses where one set of data is collected from a self-administered survey and the other is collected over the phone. Differences could emerge (or be masked) between the two groups based on differential survey methods and not differential patient satisfaction values and reactions, though research by Meterko et al. (1990) found no difference in the results generated by telephone surveying. Yet, even with this constraint, we believe that you will be a step closer to learning about the generalizability of your original respondent sample if you use this method to follow up with nonrespondents.

Please be careful because research is never a black-and-white issue. If the results of the telephone survey match all the demographics, clinical dimensions, and patient judgments and reactions to the original or mailed survey, then we are just a step closer to saying the results of the mailed survey are generalizable. The operative phrase is, "just a step closer." We have not proven, and may never be able to totally establish, the generalizability of the results of our first group of mailed survey respondents. All we have done is become a little more confident in the generalizability of these results.

One final note: Establishing the representativeness of your sample can become, in part, a statistical issue. Please rely on sound statistical and research methods consulting for this and other sampling issues.

Conclusion

Sampling, distribution, and response rates are critical issues that underlie effective patient satisfaction measurement. The best survey in the world can be reduced to meaningless proportions if the respondents are not representative of the population served and if the response rates are too small. These issues are worth spending time on because they matter a great deal in the success of any patient satisfaction measurement system.

PART IV

ANALYZING PATIENT
SATISFACTION DATA

8

MANAGING AND ANALYZING
QUANTITATIVE SURVEY DATA

The surveys are flooding in. Extra mail personnel have been hired to support the effort. The best news is that the surveys are stuffed with data. Patients are answering the vast majority of the survey questions, and they are filling the pages with qualitative comments. Now what?

Data Entry and Writing Computer
Programs to Analyze Data

The first part of this chapter focuses on ways to ensure that your data are correctly entered into a data base and that computer programs are of sufficient quality to analyze your data properly. If you are a person who tends to be obsessive and compulsive about record keeping and balancing your checkbook, then you will be at an advantage when it comes to effectively accomplishing this critical task.

Data Entry

If your data are inaccurately entered into your data base, then your patient satisfaction measurement system has been rendered useless. Here are some guidelines to prevent this from happening.

Use trained keypunchers

Trained keypunchers (data entry operators) are less likely to make systematic errors in data entry. If the keypuncher always hits the number 5 instead of hitting the number 2, then the accuracy of your system is in serious jeopardy. To further minimize the chance for such a disaster, you must continually and routinely verify the work of all your data entry operators.

Develop clear and precise coding rules

What happens when a respondent circles more than one number on the same response scale to a single survey question?

SD   D   N   A   SA

My doctor treated me with dignity and respect.   1   2   3   ④ ⑤

Should you flip a coin to decide whether you should enter a 4 or a 5 into the data base? Or should you toss out the data and enter a missing value code? Perhaps you should take the high or low score on alternative occasions?

    In this situation you should disregard the data and code the data as missing because the respondent is obviously confused if the instructions specified one choice only. Other similar rules need to be established. For instance, what if the respondent indicates that he or she waited 15–20 minutes to see the doctor? In this case, you may want to enter the midpoint—17 minutes the first time this occurs, and 18 minutes when another respondent answers the question in a similar fashion. Coding rules should be systematically defined, written down, and then reviewed for their efficacy on an ongoing basis.

Precode certain survey questions

PSMS has found it very useful to precode surveys before they are sent to the keypuncher. A trained coder reviews the survey, makes coding decisions where they need to be made, and translates dates and other data into numerical values—for example, 06/92 becomes 18 92 for the keypuncher since the survey began in January (month 01) 1991 (year 91). If names are being entered into the survey and they need to be shortened because there are not enough fields in your computer coding scheme to handle the whole name, then the precoder can make the necessary adjustments as well. For example, the name "Michelangelo di Lodovico Buonarroti Simoni" would get precoded as "Michelangelo."

Give keypunchers and coders extensive training in your system

The more the data entry operators and coders understand the big picture, the better the job they will do. They must understand the importance of their job and how misjudgments or systematic errors on their part can create serious analytical and ultimately even managerial problems.

Use sophisticated data entry software

Software currently exists that can simplify and improve the quality of your data entry. For instance, suppose we ask, "How satisfied were you with the nursing care you received?" and ask for responses on a seven-point scale. With some programs a computer "beep" will sound, signaling that an error has been made, if the data entry operator enters an impossible value, such as an 8. Some software packages (such as FOXPRO) allow the data entry operator to "paint" the actual survey on the computer screen, also serving to minimize errors.

In summary, be systematic, logical, consistent, and, most importantly, careful in designing and implementing your data management system. As significantly, remember to evaluate your system on an ongoing basis.

Computer Programs to Analyze Your Data

We shudder at the thought of how much data would be incorrectly analyzed if the computer programs analyzing the data contained mistakes. In our parlance, this would be a "fatal flaw" in survey research. Here are some rules that all patient satisfaction researchers should follow to ensure accuracy.

Do not write computer programs on your own unless you have a strong programming background

Hire someone who is trained in using any of the excellent data base management and statistical software packages on the market. Examples include FOXPRO, DBASE IV, SPSS (Statistical Package for Social Sciences) or SAS (the Statistical Analysis System). Doing this yourself would be analogous to rebuilding your automobile's automatic transmission. It takes time, patience, intense verification, and training to correctly write these programs and maintain them over time.

Make sure the computer programmer validates his or her programs

We cannot overemphasize how important validation is. There are many ways it can be done. Typically, the more different ways a program is validated, the safer you will be.

Just because a program is validated doesn't mean that you can sleep well for the rest of your life. Programs should be validated each time a new data set is brought up on a monthly or quarterly basis. The time it takes to validate a program is never so excessive that it is not worth the effort.

Prepare a detailed code book

A code book in survey research is like a libretto in opera: It tells you what is happening. A sample of a PSMS code book is shown in Exhibit 8.1. The accuracy of the code book must be as meticulously managed as the accuracy of your computer programming and data entry.

Code books serve another very useful purpose: They help the end user of the data to understand what the computer output results mean. For many people, much of the work mentioned above can be quite tedious, like balancing your checkbook or doing your taxes. However, it would be far worse to have to tell your boss that you were slipshod in your data management methods and that all the data you have reported to him or her for the last six months happens to be just a little wrong!

Analyzing Your Data

Accuracy of Data

Our PSMS team at the Ohio State University's College of Medicine strongly believes in this motto: Assume that your data are wrong until proven otherwise. Although this is the opposite of how the American legal system operates, it is the foundation of a solid data base management program. The reason we believe in this motto is that we have found it to be true, at least to some extent. That is why the first step in data analysis is to reverify that your data have been correctly keypunched and that your computer programs are accurately written.

Step 1

Study the distribution of values that your respondents have assigned to the items in your survey. Ask yourself the following questions:

- Is it possible to have length of stays equaling 0 days or exceeding 245 days? This is called *range check analysis*.
- Is it possible that 81 percent of the respondents came from our oncology service? I thought Health Hospital had only five oncology beds? This is called *logic check analysis*.

- Is it possible to have two survey identification numbers that are the same? This is called *being thorough*.

The results of every survey item must be scrutinized in this manner to ensure accuracy.

Step 2

Like a good detective, you should verify any questionable data input, going back to the original surveys and computer programs.

Step 3

Ask your programmer to write subroutines that will flag outliers and illogical relationships that may exist in your data base.

Descriptive Analysis

Descriptive analysis involves generating the following kinds of statistics: mean (the average score), mode (the single score respondents most frequently assign), median (the value in the distribution of scores where half the scores are higher than that number and the other half of the scores are lower), standard deviation (the degree of spread or variation of all the scores), and range (the lowest value and the highest value).

Standard deviation

In reviewing these scores, be sensitive to the standard deviation—how spread out or densely packed all respondents' scores are. Suppose that on the survey question "My nurses responded to my calls for assistance quickly. SD D N A SA," 98 percent of the respondents answer SA, resulting in an extremely small standard deviation. The health care manager now has a difficult choice between two alternatives:

1. Is this question insensitive to differences (variation) in patient perceptions of "call responsiveness"?
2. Or is this question actually generating valid information, and in this sample virtually all the nurses are terrific in their responsiveness to patient calls for help?

Ultimately, it becomes a judgment call. However, the fact that 98 percent of the respondents answered only one value (SA) should make one question the validity, if not the usefulness, of the item.

Exhibit 8.1 Code Book Example

DIRECTIONS

Please respond to each question by circling the number or checking the box that best describes your experience during your most recent stay at The Health Hospital. If any question does **NOT APPLY** to you, please leave it blank.

Scale: SD = Strongly Disagree, **D** = Disagree, **N** = Neither Agree Nor Disagree, **A** = Agree, **SA** = Strongly Agree.

PREADMISSION

1 Was this your first hospitalization at The Health Hospital? .... ☐ Yes ☐ No

I1 C22

2 How many times have you been hospitalized in the past 12 months?

_____ Hospitalizations

I2 C23–24

3 Parking was *not* a problem. SD D N A SA

I3 C25

4 The system of signs made it easy for me to find my way around the hospital. .... SD D N A SA

I4 C26

ADMISSIONS

1 How were you admitted to The Health Hospital? (check **ALL** that apply)

A. As a patient from The Health Hospital's Emergency Department .... ☐ Yes ☐ No

I5 C27

B. From another hospital (transfer) ... ☐ Yes ☐ No

I6 C28

C. For Labor and Delivery .... ☐ Yes ☐ No

I7 C29

D. Sent directly to Surgery <u>before</u> going to your room .... ☐ Yes ☐ No

I8 C30

E. Pre-planned or Scheduled Admission .... ☐ Yes ☐ No

I9 C31

2 The admitting staff was:

Courteous .... SD D N A SA   I10 C32

Responsive .... SD D N A SA   I11 C33

3 The admitting process was
handled efficiently. .... SD D N A SA   I12 C34

4 The amount of time between
when you arrived at the
hospital until you went to
your room was acceptable. .... SD D N A SA   I13 C35

Approximately, how long was it? _____ Minutes   I14 C36–38

5 If you had to wait, did the
admitting staff keep you
updated on how long your
wait would be?   □ Yes   □ No   □ Did not wait   I15 C39

Comments on Admissions: _____

_____

ENVIRONMENT AND FOOD

1 My room was:

Clean	SD	D	N	A	SA	I16 C40
Comfortable	SD	D	N	A	SA	I17 C41
Quiet	SD	D	N	A	SA	I18 C42
Well Maintained	SD	D	N	A	SA	I19 C43

2 Overall, I found the hospital environment to be:

Clean	SD	D	N	A	SA	I20 C44
Comfortable	SD	D	N	A	SA	I21 C45
Friendly	SD	D	N	A	SA	I22 C46
Homey	SD	D	N	A	SA	I23 C47

3 The food was appetizing,
considering my dietary
restrictions. .... SD D N A SA   I24 C48

4 The appearance of the food
was appealing. .... SD D N A SA   I25 C49

5 My meals were served at the
appropriate temperature. .... SD D N A SA   I26 C50

6 The nutrition service's staff
explained my diet and menu
restrictions thoroughly. .... SD D N A SA   I27 C51

7 The people who delivered my meal trays were:

Courteous	SD	D	N	A	SA	I28 C52
Responsive	SD	D	N	A	SA	I29 C53

Comments on Environment and Food: _____

_____

Note: I = variable name; C = column number.

Average scores and median scores

Aside from the standard deviation, the average score will probably be the descriptive statistic on which you will rely most heavily. The mean, or average, will summarize in a single value how respondents in general felt about a given issue. However, the mean or average score can be very deceiving, as the following example will show.

Suppose you asked patients how long it took for them to get from admitting to their rooms, and the results of your sample looked like Table 8.1. How well does the average reflect what is truly occurring in the data? The answer is, not very well. Two outliers (patients 3 and 8) are dramatically raising the overall average. Hence, the median will be a more accurate representation of the respondents' scores. In this case, the median is 33 minutes. When the two outliers are excluded from the data, the average waiting time for 82 percent of this sample is reduced to 29 minutes! With waiting time data, in particular, and other variables where a few outlier values can distort your average score (for example, length of stay), the median is the statistic of choice.

Average scores can be deceiving in another similar way. Suppose one of the items was "Parking was not a problem," and the results looked like Table 8.2. In these data, the average score may be considered acceptable. Although not a score over 4.00, 3.58 suggests that all is not bad with parking. However, more than the mean should always be investigated by the health care manager. Closer inspection of these data suggest that there is a bipolar

Table 8.1 Sample Survey of Time It Took to Get to Room

Case ID	Waiting Time (minutes)
1	20
2	12
3	240
4	21
5	36
6	33
7	17
8	300
9	23
10	46
11	53

Average waiting time = 72.82 minutes

Table 8.2 Sample Results to "Parking Was Not a Problem"

	Assigned Value	*Frequency*	*Percent*
Strongly Disagree	1	48	19.1
Disagree	2	9	3.6
Neither Agree/Disagree	3	8	3.2
Agree	4	121	48.2
Strongly Agree	5	65	25.9
Totals		251	100%

Average Score = 3.58

distribution—many respondents are indeed happy with parking (about 74 percent answered Strongly Agree or Agree), yet over 22 percent, a sizeable proportion, are unhappy with parking, assigning answers of Strongly Disagree or Disagree. If the health care manager is not careful, the mean may mask the presence of this problem group.

The message to health care managers is clear: Always look at your response distributions and standard deviation in addition to your mean and median.

Beware of positive response set bias

A second phenomenon to be sensitive to is *positive response set bias*, also known as *leniency effects*. Patient satisfaction research typically shows that patients tend to give high (positive) scores, especially when evaluating their health care providers. Reasons for this, cited earlier, include the unwillingness to be critical of one's health care providers and the respondent's desire to say the "right thing." Of particular note is that some patients will choose to decline to answer a question rather than make a critical remark about the hospital or a provider. Hence, when a respondent declines to answer a survey item, we believe it is safe to assume that the patient is more likely to be withholding a critical assessment than a positive one. This, too, will contribute to the upward biasing we tend to see in patient satisfaction scores.

Building Overall Indicator Scores

One of the best ways to analyze patient satisfaction data is through the construction of *overall indicator scores*. Overall indicator scores involve combining the respondents' answers to conceptually similar types of questions and then summarizing them as a single value. Consider the example shown in Table 8.3 to better understand this idea better.

In this example, average scores for each nursing care item are calculated. However, an overall indicator score also can be created to summarize, in a single value, all four nursing care items.

To accomplish this, we create a new composite variable for each separate respondent called Nursing Care

$$\text{Nursing care overall indicator score} = \frac{(\text{Sensitive} + \text{Caring} + \text{Friendly} + \text{Empathetic})}{4}$$

Note that this is not the average score of the four item averages listed in Table 8.3. Instead, a separate nursing care indicator average score for each respondent is first calculated, as shown in Table 8.4. If the respondent has missing data on any of the four variables comprising the overall indicator score, then an overall indicator score is not computed for this person. Subsequently, these individual average scores are averaged across all the respondents to generate an overall nursing care indicator average score.

Table 8.3   Health Hospital Survey Questions On Nursing Care

My Nurses Were	SD	D	N	A	SA	Average	Cases
Sensitive	1	2	3	4	5	3.21	322
Caring	1	2	3	4	5	2.92	345
Friendly	1	2	3	4	5	3.87	315
Empathetic	1	2	3	4	5	3.45	334

Table 8.4   Data for Each Respondent for Survey Questions on Nursing Care

	Sensitive	Caring	Friendly	Empathetic	Average Individual Score
Respondent 1	4	3	4	3	3.50
Respondent 2	1	2	2	1	1.50
Respondent 3	3	3	5	4	3.75
Respondent 4	2	3	2	3	2.50
Overall nursing care indicator average score					2.81

There are a number of advantages and risks to using overall indicator scores. We will begin by exploring some of the advantages.

First, by creating overall indicator scores we are reducing the amount of data with which the health care manager must work. One score is easier to understand than four scores.

Second, this approach allows health care managers to view these data on two levels—the individual item level and the combined overall indicator score level. The manager can identify which individual survey items are causing the overall indicator score to rise and which are causing it to fall. In a sense, the overall indicator score becomes the *what*, and the specific survey items comprising it become the *why* behind the *what*.

In Table 8.5, data are displayed on dietary staff attitudes and behaviors as evaluated by patients. From these data, the health care manager can identify which items are raising the overall dietary indicator score and which are lowering it. If the manager is going to try to improve this score over time, he or she would be wise to allocate some thought, energy, and perhaps resources to improving the promptness of dietary services.

There are at least four risks to computing overall indicator scores that should be noted. First, they may encourage the health care manager to become dependent solely on the overall indicator score and not bother to look at the results of items that create this score. In this instance, the manager is only looking at the *what* and never investigating the equally or more important question, *why*.

Table 8.5 Sample Data for Survey Questions on Dietary Staff

$$\text{Overall dietary staff indicator score} = \frac{\left(\begin{array}{l}\text{Dietary staff was prompt in delivering services}\end{array} + \begin{array}{l}\text{Dietary staff explained my dietary restrictions to me}\end{array} + \begin{array}{l}\text{Dietary staff was courteous to me}\end{array}\right)}{3}$$

	Average	Cases
Overall dietary staff indicator score	4.12	541
Diet staff prompt	3.61	562
Diet staff explained	4.32	543
Diet staff courteous	4.41	546

Note: Five-point scale where 1 = Strongly Disagree and 5 = Strongly Agree.

Second, the internal reliability of the indicator score may not be acceptable, so the overall indicator score should not be used to summarize the group of items. The health care manager should consult with statisticians and ask them to generate the *Cronbach alpha reliability statistic*, adjusted for the number of items that comprise the overall indicator score.

Third, the overall indicator score may be comprised of items that do not conceptually fit together—the proverbial "apples and oranges" problem. The items comprising overall indicator scores should have a common conceptual theme. Aggregating nursing satisfaction items with physician satisfaction items, for example, would not make sense. The health care manager should also consult with a statistician to evaluate this issue statistically, through a technique called *factor analysis*.

A fourth concern is missing data. If the individual items making up the overall indicator score have too much missing data, then the overall score could be misleading. For example, suppose the overall indicator score for billing satisfaction and the individual item scores that comprise it look like Table 8.6.

In this example, there are 339 missing cases for the variable "billing was accurate," and no missing cases for the variable "billing was understandable." Aggregating the data in the way we recommend would mean that 339 cases of the second item would not be used in the calculation of the overall billing satisfaction indicator score. The concern is that we are throwing out a lot of data by using the missing data exclusion rule discussed earlier. In instances where the number of cases comprising the overall indicator score is widely variant, the patient satisfaction researcher should seriously consider not calculating the overall indicator score. Another alternative is to calculate what is called a *weighted average* overall indicator score; however, you should consult with a knowledgeable statistician to understand the costs and benefits of this. A concern with weighted averaging is that we are giving a

Table 8.6   Overall Satisfaction with Billing Indicator Score and Specific Items (Sample Size = 550)

	Average	*Cases*
Overall satisfaction with billing	2.92	211
Billing accurate	2.21	211
Billing understandable	3.62	550

Note: Five-point scale where 1 = Strongly Disagree and 5 = Strongly Agree.

single item more or less influence on the overall indicator score based on sample size rather than basing the weighting scheme on sound theory.

Breakdown Analysis

The concept

Earlier we discussed what was referred to as the "unit-of-analysis problem." We noted that patient satisfaction measurement systems are no better than your ability to break down your data into smaller groups.

For instance, to know that the overall indicator score for nursing services is 4.32 on a five-point scale is helpful, but also terribly limiting. What do you do with that number? What *can* you do with that number? The answer is, very little, unless you can break down your data into smaller groups (units of analysis), such as nursing discharge unit, DRG, medical service, admitting physician, in order to generate practical and useful information. That is why so much time must be spent on designing and implementing the label-encoding process described in Chapter 3.

The model

Figure 8.1 displays a breakdown model. You should pay special attention to three aspects of the model:

1. Begin data analysis at the overall hospital or outpatient level.
2. Always incorporate overall indicator score analysis with individual item analysis.
3. The unit of analysis becomes increasingly more specific as one progresses through the model.

Table 8.7 is an example of how the first level of analysis for a total health care organization might be presented. The overall indicator scores and standard deviations (not included) should be shown, followed by the specific item averages that comprise the overall indicator scores. Additionally, some basic demographic and clinical data about your survey population should be included—for instance, what percent of the respondents were male/female and average age of respondents.

Table 8.8 is an example of the next level of analysis that the health care manager should conduct. Data broken down by nursing discharge unit will give the health care manager much more detailed and operationally useful information than only hospitalwide data. The health care manager can discern from Table 8.8 that nursing unit 2 West may be having difficulty

Figure 8.1 A Conceptual Model for Breaking Down
Patient Satisfaction Survey Results into
Meaningful Groupings

First Level: Sublevel 1

Overall health care
organizational analysis

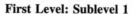

Second Level: Sublevels 2 to 5

Analyses by nursing unit, attending physician, or DRG,
dietary, medical service, demographics

Third Level: Sublevel 7

Multidimensional breakdowns
Cross-analyses (such as
satisfaction with dietary staff)
broken down by nursing discharge staff

"listening" to their patients. This could indicate poor listening skills among staff, very sick patients, inadequate staffing, or other factors.

When reviewing the data from 3 East, the health care manager must be careful not to jump to any premature conclusions, because only 16 discharged patients from this nursing discharge unit responded to the survey. Statistics based on small sample sizes should be viewed with *extreme caution.*

These data are presented as unadjusted scores; that is, no patient-mix adjustment has been made to these scores (see the following section). There is nothing wrong with this; however, drawing comparative conclusions (for example, between nursing units) based on these data should not be done until patient-mix adjustment has been made. For example, one unit's scores may be higher or lower on a given item because of their average patient age or acuity and not because their nurses performed any better or worse than another unit's nurses on that particular item.

Table 8.7 First Level of Analysis—Subhead 1: Overall Health Care Organizational Level

- Analyze overall indicator scores
- Analyze the items that comprise each overall indicator scores

Overall Indicator Scores and Individual Item Scores	Average Score	Cases
Satisfaction with physicians	3.44	632
Doctors listened	2.84	632
Doctors explained	3.97	632
Doctors cared	3.51	632
Satisfaction with preadmitting	3.60	622
Forms readable	3.21	622
Information was clearly presented	3.98	622
Information was helpful	3.61	622
Satisfaction with parking (single item measure)	2.12	598
Satisfaction with food quality	4.77	598
Food served hot	4.91	598
Food appealing	4.62	598
Food as ordered	4.77	598

Note: Five-point scale where 1 = Strongly Disagree and 5 = Strongly Agree.

Finally, be sensitive to the accuracy of the label. Unless otherwise controlled for, some patients who were transferred may be commenting on nursing services they received in intensive care, or even the emergency department. This potential confound and suggested ways of managing it are discussed back in Chapter 4.

The second level of analysis, sublevel 3, breaks down the data by medical service (Table 8.9). This information will not only be of particular interest to the health care manager but also to the medical director and the medical staff. Again, be very careful about drawing any conclusions until the sample size has been deemed sufficiently large and the standard deviations associated with each mean score are considered (not shown in Table 8.9). Moreover, drawing conclusions about why the scores from one service are higher or lower than another should again not be made until the scores

Table 8.8 Second Level of Analysis—Sublevel 2: Data Broken Down by Nursing Discharge Unit

- Analyze overall indicator scores
- Analyze the items that comprise overall indicator scores
- Analyze other pertinent items

	Average Scores				
	3E	*3W*	*2E*	*2W*	*All Nursing Units*
Overall nursing satisfaction indicator score	4.17	4.05	3.85	3.53	4.04
Nurses listened	4.89	3.92	3.67	2.98	
Nurses explained	4.12	3.81	3.87	3.41	
Nurses cared	3.51	4.43	4.00	4.21	

Note: Five-point scale where 1 = Strongly Disagree and 5 = Strongly Agree. Average number of respondents per nursing discharge unit is 56. Nursing discharge unit 2E has only 16 discharges who returned patient satisfaction survey data. The overall mean of 4.04 is due to the large number of cases in 3W relative to the other nursing units.

Table 8.9 Second Level of Analysis—Sublevel 3: Data Broken Down by Medical Service

- Analyze overall indicator scores
- Analyze the items that comprise each overall indicator score
- Analyze other pertinent items

	Ob/Gyn	*Medicine*	*Surgery*	*Pediatrics*	*All Services*
Overall satisfaction indicator scores for physicians	3.55	3.63	3.85	4.06	3.77
Doctors listened	2.89	2.98	2.67	3.32	2.97
Doctors explained	4.32	4.25	4.87	4.12	4.39
Doctors cared	3.43	3.65	4.01	4.76	3.96

Note: Five-point scale where 1 = Strongly Disagree and 5 = Strongly Agree. Complete data; no missing cases.

have been patient-mix adjusted. Even then, such conclusions should only be drawn with great care.

Note that many variables/items could be broken down by medical service beyond "overall satisfaction with physician care." For instance, overall indicator scores on satisfaction with nursing care or room, and the items comprising these overall indicator scores, could be easily analyzed by medical service.

In Table 8.10, consistent with our analytical plan, the level of analysis has become more specific: The data have been broken down by individual

Table 8.10   Second Level of Analysis—Sublevel 4: Data Broken Down by Attending Physician (or DRG)

- Analyze overall indicator scores
- Analyze the items that comprise each overall indicator score
- Analyze other pertinent items

Medical Identification Number	*Average Score*	*Cases*
M.D. #132 overall indicator score	3.44	339
M.D. told me what was happening to me	3.56	351
M.D. clearly answered all of my questions	3.61	356
M.D. demonstrated sensitivity to me as a patient	3.21	340
M.D. #243 overall indicator score	4.12	140
M.D. told me what was happening to me	4.41	149
M.D. clearly answered all of my questions	3.91	147
M.D. demonstrated sensitivity to me as a patient	4.04	150
M.D. #456 overall indicator score	3.02	152
M.D. told me what was happening to me	3.03	167
M.D. clearly answered all of my questions	3.00	171
M.D. demonstrated sensitivity to me as a patient	3.02	170
M.D. #496 overall indicator score	4.54	201
M.D. told me what was happening to me	4.78	221
M.D. clearly answered all of my questions	4.32	219
M.D. demonstrated sensitivity to me as a patient	4.53	211

Note: Five-point scale where 1 = Strongly Disagree and 5 = Strongly Agree.

physician (admitting or discharge, depending on how your encoded label is designed). Again, one could look at many other variables, such as "willingness to return to this health care organization for medical care," "willingness to recommend," or "overall satisfaction with inpatient stay," broken down by DRG, medical diagnostic category, or ICD-9 codes. The caveats pertaining to making comparisons raised earlier should be kept in mind at this level of analysis, too. In addition, one must take care to ensure that the physician identification number on the encoded label will correspond to the physician the patient is referring to when he or she completes the survey (see Chapters 4 and 5 for a detailed discussion of this potential confound).

Further breakdown analysis can be conducted using the demographic data included on the encoded label. In the example in Table 8.11, the health care manager is investigating gender differences in the perceptions of physician care. In this hypothetical example, females were more satisfied than males with the overall care provided by their physician. An important reason for this difference seems to come from the items "the doctors cared" and "the doctors listened." Again, be cautious of between-group comparisons if patient-mix adjustment has not been conducted.

The third level of analysis, sublevel 6, represents the most detailed and specific unit of analysis. In the example in Table 8.12, the health care

Table 8.11   Second Level of Analysis—Sublevel 5: Data Broken Down by Sex (or Age, Month or Quarter of Discharge, and Other Demographic Variables)

- Analyze overall indicator scores
- Analyze the items that comprise each overall indicator score
- Analyze other pertinent items

	Males (n = 349)	*Females* (n = 421)	*Statistically Significant* (p < .05)?
Overall satisfaction indicator scores for physicians	3.54	4.18	Yes
Doctors listened	2.89	3.86	Yes
Doctors explained	4.32	4.25	No
Doctors cared	3.43	4.43	Yes

Note: Five-point scale where 1 = Strongly Disagree and 5 = Strongly Agree.

manager is looking at patient satisfaction with physicians broken down by gender and then further broken down by medical service. The manager has learned that both men and women rate "medicine" higher on the physician satisfaction overall indicator score and items than "surgery." In addition, men rate "medicine" and "surgery" higher than women. Patient-mix adjustment should be conducted on these scores if possible.

The number of multidimensional breakdowns is virtually limitless, presenting both a blessing and curse. It is a blessing because we can break down the data to answer virtually any patient satisfaction research question that we desire. It is a curse because the patient satisfaction researcher and health care manager can easily get engulfed in an endless quagmire of data and computer outputs. We recommend thinking through exactly the kind of questions you wish to answer before having the computer generate 1,000 multidimensional breakdown analyses.

Breakdown analysis is the heart of excellent analytical schemes of patient satisfaction measurement systems for both quantitative and qualitative analyses. The quality and specificity of feedback generated through this basic analytical tool can, theoretically, pay large operational dividends.

Table 8.12 Third Level of Analysis—Sublevel 6: Multidimensional Breakdowns

- For example, satisfaction with dietary services broken down by medical service and nursing discharge unit
- Satisfaction with physicians broken down by medical service, nursing discharge unit, etc.

	Average Scores			
	Males (n = 306)		Females (n = 391)	
	Medicine	Surgery	Medicine	Surgery
Overall satisfaction indicator scores for physicians	4.77	3.21	4.41	3.03
Doctors listened	4.88	3.20	4.81	2.78
Doctors explained	4.76	3.22	4.02	3.33
Doctors cared	4.69	3.23	4.42	2.99

Note: Between-gender comparisons for medicine and surgery combined are statistically significant at $p < .05$. Between-service comparisons across gender are statistically significant at $p < .05$.

Patient-Mix Adjustment and Comparisons

A hypothetical scenario

We are implementing a patient satisfaction measurement program in a three-hospital system: Hospital A, Hospital B, and Hospital C. We know from analyzing the data from this hospital system that sicker patients tend to be less satisfied with a variety of services and providers than less sick patients. This relationship appears in all three hospitals. Assume that Hospital A has a much higher acuity index than either Hospital B or C. Originally, however, management at the ABC hospital system was not aware of the relationship to patient satisfaction scores. Nevertheless, a patient satisfaction survey was conducted and the data Table 8.13 emerged.

Table 8.13   Overall Satisfaction with Stay: The ABC Hospital System (Unadjusted Scores)

	Average Score	Standard Deviation	Cases
Hospital A	2.67	1.11	434
Hospital B	4.12	1.02	245
Hospital C	4.32	1.07	323
Overall	3.56*		1,002

Note: Five-point scale where 1 = Strongly Disagree and 5 = Strongly Agree.
*Weighted average.

When corporate management received these data they asked the CEO at Hospital A the obvious question, "Why are your scores so low?" Mary Davidson, the CEO for Hospital A, replied, "The reasons our scores are so low is that we treat much sicker patients." She went on to show how all the differences in hospital satisfaction scores could be accounted for by patient acuity. When the numbers are adjusted for patient acuity, Davidson's Hospital A comes out smelling like a rose. When the adjusted data analysis is run, the results look like Table 8.14.

The next generation of patient satisfaction measurement will begin to rely on patient-mix adjustment so that more meaningful and fairer interdepartment, inter–medical service, and interhospital comparisons can be made. Patient age and patient acuity are two of many potential factors that you might consider adjusting for in your data analysis format. Without statistically adjusting for factors that can influence patient satisfaction ratings, it

Table 8.14 Overall Satisfaction with Stay: The ABC Hospital System (Adjusted for Acuity)

	Average Score	*Standard Deviation*	*Cases*
Hospital A	3.98	1.11	434
Hospital B	3.54	1.02	245
Hospital C	3.31	1.07	323
Overall	3.56*		

Note: Five-point scale where 1 = Strongly Disagree and 5 = Strongly Agree.
*Weighted average.

is all too easy to formulate inaccurate conclusions about why high and low scores exist. The Mary Davidson tale is an example of this.

The challenge of patient-mix adjustment is largely statistical. Hence, health care managers should rely on statistical consulting help, either in-house (perhaps through their marketing department) or from an outside source.

Does this mean that unadjusted data are absolutely useless? No, it simply means that you have to be much more cautious in interpreting and drawing conclusions from your comparative data. Certainly noncomparative analyses can be made without concern for patient-mix adjustment. However, this may limit the usefulness of your data.

What Is a Good Score?

Of all the questions we are asked about data analysis, "What is a good score?" is probably the most frequently asked. As frustrating as it may be to health care managers, we can only offer rough guidelines.

Why the ambiguity? Because the answer depends on so many factors:

1. What are management's expectations?

2. What are the norms, and are they accurate?

3. Have the scores been patient-mix adjusted?

4. How does a given score look in the context of what has been going on in the health care organization?

5. What value judgments are managers bringing to the score interpretation table?

6. How are the survey items written, and what do they truly measure?

With all of this ambiguity and uncertainty in mind, we present the following guidelines, albeit with some trepidation.

Guideline 1: Absolute values for five- and ten-point scales

On a five-point scale, scores of 4.25 and above may signal excellence; scores of 4.00 and better usually indicate that things are alright; scores below 4.00 might suggest that the manager follow up to assess if a problem is present. For ten-point scales, which should not be used that often, scores of 8.5 and above may signal excellence. Scores between 8.1 and 8.49 may indicate that things are alright. Scores 8 and below should raise some concern. Our experience with seven-point scales is too limited to make any kind of similar recommendation.

Guideline 2: Use the anchors on your scales

Consider a previous example from this chapter: the item "Parking was not a problem" (Table 8.2). The "agreement/disagreement" anchors on the survey scale tell us a great deal about what is good and what is not. For instance, it is good that over 74 percent of the respondents scored Agree or Strongly Agree on this item, though one might wish for an even higher percentage. It is not good that 19 percent scored Strongly Disagree. Scales that are anchored with Excellent, Good, Average, Fair, and Poor can give the health care manager information on the absolute quality or value of a score as well.

Guideline 3: Use norms, though with care

Norms are an acceptable way to assess what is a good score. However, make sure the norms are current (for example, not ten years old) and that they are derived from similar institutions serving similar patient populations. Beware of percentile differences that have very little meaning in absolute terms. For instance, suppose you are told that your overall physician satisfaction indicator score is in the 80th percentile. If the 95th percentile is only .15 higher on a five-point scale (4.35 compared to 4.50), then the 80th percentile means very little in absolute value terms.

In general, we do believe in the use and value of norms. However, it seems that too much emphasis has been placed on them in the past. We believe that the best norm you have is your own hospital's or outpatient clinic's patient satisfaction scores longitudinally trended over time.

Guideline 4: The best indicator of a good or a bad score is generated by tracking your health care organization over time

Patient satisfaction measurement systems that track their scores over time will get the best idea of what a good score is, because the best comparison group of all is your own hospital or outpatient clinic compared to itself over time.

If you start with an overall dietary satisfaction indicator score of 3.47, and within four quarters it goes to 3.98, then that's certainly a very good score. This is not to say that more improvement in dietary isn't needed. However, it does focus on the most important way to use state-of-the-art patient satisfaction measurement: as a tool for improving the quality of care and services rendered!

Other Data Analysis Tips

1. There are many other data analytic procedures that can (and should) be applied to help you better understand your data: for example, t-tests, chi-square analysis, regression analysis, and causal model building. These are powerful analytical tools that should be employed. Consulting with a trained statistician will be needed to apply these statistical procedures and interpret the ensuing analyses appropriately.

2. Be very careful of making inaccurate causal attributions. Suppose you find that a given nursing unit's overall nursing satisfaction indicator score has been very low for four consecutive months. Some health care managers would have a tendency to point fingers and assign blame to those "lazy, indifferent, overpaid nurses." Do not do this until you have all the facts. The score could be explained by a host of alternative hypotheses, such as higher patient acuity, severe staffing shortages, older or younger patients, or an awful day/afternoon shift supervisor.

3. Use other data to confirm or disconfirm your interpretations. Patient satisfaction measurement represents only one manner in which evaluations can be made. What health care providers and managers observe and hear are equally important perspectives to consider.

4. Be very careful of making interpretations when you are dealing with small sample sizes.

5. Know who your respondents are so that you can assess the generalizability of your survey results.

6. Avoid getting swamped by all the data you generate. The proverbial "forest and trees" problem is all too likely to emerge if you lose sight of what you are attempting to accomplish.

7. Know the limitations of your data set. For instance, has patient-mix adjustment been made? Are there a lot of missing data in your data set? Are only older patients responding to the survey? Are the data on the encoded label matching those people whom the patients are referring to in their survey responses? You will not be representing your data properly unless you are aware of the data's limitations and you also report them. All patient satisfaction measurement systems, and the data sets they generate, have limitations.

8. Take your time reviewing your data. Although today's health care managers are indeed crunched for time, if you rush through the analysis and interpretation of your patient satisfaction data, you are reducing the potential effectiveness of a very potent tool.

9. Be careful to ensure the accuracy of your data.

10. Back up your data on an ongoing basis. Have it located in more than one geographical location.

11. Be conservative in your interpretations! It is all too easy to get carried away with your data and begin to make statements and draw conclusions that may not be accurate or fair.

Conclusion

Quantitative data must be analyzed with great care and forethought. The information is powerful, and it can be all too easily misused. Remember, too, that it is limited: It represents only one method of assessing patient satisfaction. Just because your quantitative data are neatly printed out on computer paper does not mean that you have envisioned the single, blinding truth. In health care there are many truths that must be considered before any final evaluation is made or conclusion is drawn.

9

MANAGING AND ANALYZING QUALITATIVE DATA

The great strides in patient satisfaction research in the next decade are likely to be made in the collection and analysis of qualitative data. The patients' written comments, as noted throughout this book, often contain the most useful and insightful evaluative information for the patient satisfaction researcher and the health care manager. The utility of patient satisfaction measurement grows dramatically when systematic qualitative analysis is conducted.

The goal of this chapter is to move health care managers and patient satisfaction researchers beyond the basic methodology of just reading or just typing a list of qualitative comments. Although there is nothing wrong with these approaches per se, there is much more that can be done to turn qualitative data into truly useful information.

Developing a Qualitative Analysis Coding Scheme

Suppose you work in a large hospital or outpatient clinic and you have been assigned the task of reading all the written comments on the returned patient satisfaction surveys. The first thing you will learn is that this is no small chore. Patients write literally all over their surveys. Health care consumers often need to communicate about their medical experiences, and the patient satisfaction survey is an excellent vehicle for giving them a sense of catharsis. Think for a moment of all the people you have heard discussing their most recent hospital stay or outpatient visit with substantial emotion. It is no secret that one's personal health care experience is a "top ten" (perhaps "top one") life event. This is a primary reason patients write extensive comments on their surveys.

The second thing you will notice in reviewing qualitative comments is that you will have trouble getting a handle on all of these data. Qualitative comments do not lend themselves to an easy-to-interpret, single overall indicator score, as we are able to generate in the quantitative measurement area. You may ask yourself: How can I make sense out of all of these comments?

The answer is to develop a qualitative analysis coding scheme—a method of categorizing all of the written comments into logical and similar groups, permitting easier understanding and interpretation of the patients' written comments. Stated differently, it is a method of reducing your data to more manageable and understandable proportions.

Designing Qualitative Coding Scheme Categories

There is no "one right" or "one best" qualitative coding scheme. The coding scheme you devise should be built around the following principles.

Your coding scheme should be easy to use

If your coding scheme is too complex, you are more likely to generate unreliable results or to ignore qualitative coding and analysis altogether. Clear-cut decision rules on categorization of written comments are critical.

Group data into a format usable by managers

Coding schemes can be constructed around a variety of dimensions. Some are probably going to be more useful for health care managers than others. For instance, as an academic, I might be very interested in coding all comments along a psychological dimension, such as "personal control" (Greenberger and Strasser 1986). I might read every patient's comment and then code each one into one of the following coding categories:

MC code = Patient's comment indicates a desire for more personal control over his or her health care outcomes.

SC code = Patient's comment indicates a possession of sufficient personal control over his or her health care outcomes.

TMC code = Patient's comment indicates that a desire for less personal control over his or her health care outcomes.

        NC code = Cannot determine from patient's comment if personal
        control issues are being expressed.

However, this kind of coding scheme probably does little to help managers do their jobs better. The key, then, is to develop a conceptual model or logical framework that allows you to turn your qualitative data into useful information.

Follow the rule of mutual exclusivity

Successful qualitative coding schemes are based on coding categories that are at right angles to one another: Coding categories should not overlap with one another. A comment that is coded into coding category A should not also be a logical fit for category B.

Be as comprehensive as is operationally possible

The coding scheme you devise should be comprehensive enough to success-fully categorize comments that comprise the full range of patients' health care experiences, exposure to stimuli, value judgments, and reactions. How-ever, if we have too many first-level categories (refer to the next section for further clarification), the system becomes unwieldy and, perhaps, more unreliable. If we have too few first-level categories, we may be back al-most to where we began—in need of finding a way to reduce our data to more manageable and understandable proportions. From our experience we have found that a good rule of thumb is to generate no more than 12 to 15 first-level categories.

Permit further categorization within each of the major categories

Further categorization is called *second-level categorization*. Suppose we have a first-level category called Admitting, which contains patients' com-ments on their admission into the health care facility (Figure 9.1). The qualitative coder may now wish to create a set of admitting subcategories. For example, the coder could break down the admitting comments into Pos-itive, Negative, and Neutral value judgments, or various kinds of reactions, such as Satisfied, Dissatisfied, Angry, Sad, Frightened, and Secure.

    Third-level categorization (and beyond) is also possible. Using the above example we might break down the Positive, Neutral, and Nega-tive admitting comments into two more third-level subcategories: comments on waiting time and comments on admitting staff behavior and attitudes (Figure 9.1).

Figure 9.1   Sample Categorization of "Admitting"

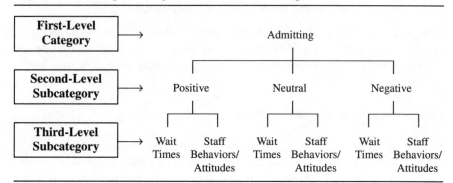

Create clear coding rules

Coders must know why one comment is coded a "nursing" comment and why another is coded a "medical treatment" comment. Hence, the designer of your coding scheme must define each category and explain why a given comment belongs there versus elsewhere. Precise examples of the kind of written comments that fall into each category should be provided. Examples should include both correct coding decisions and commonly made coding errors to be avoided. Guidelines must be provided for what coders should do if they are uncertain about a coding decision. What to do with anomalies should also be discussed. The end product should be a code book, where all of these rules, guidelines, and protocols are incorporated. Coders need to be carefully trained in how to accurately conduct qualitative coding. The training also needs to be ongoing because it is easy to form bad coding habits.

All this may sound pretty straightforward, but it's not. It is very difficult to develop, implement, and maintain an excellent qualitative coding scheme. This is one main reason why thorough qualitative analysis has been historically avoided. The following example is provided to show how difficult qualitative coding can be.

Suppose that you only have the following first-level coding categories available to you:

- Nursing comments
- Physician comments
- Medical treatment comments
- Miscellaneous comments
- Medical students (first- through fourth-year students only)

In addition, you have second-level categories (within each first-level category): Positive Comments, Negative Comments, and Neutral Comments. A patient's completed survey is received. On the back of her survey under the section "General Comments," she writes:

> The doctors and nurses were terrific except for the one resident who was really rude to me. My other concern was that the doctor did not conduct an echocardiogram for me like other doctors have in the past.

How should this be coded? Should the phrase "doctors . . . were terrific" be coded as a Physician Positive comment, or does the medical resident's rudeness offset this and hence you code nothing (a negative washes out a positive)? Perhaps, the phrase "doctors . . . were terrific" should be coded as a Physician Positive comment, while the resident's rudeness should be coded as a Physician Negative comment? And this brings to mind another question: Is a resident a "physician" or a "medical student"? What about the nurses? Should the phrase "doctors and nurses were terrific" be coded twice (double-coded)—one comment for the Physician Positive category and one for the Nursing Positive category—or should we code this comment into the Other Positive category? How about the echocardiogram? Should this be coded as a Physician Negative comment or should it be coded as a Medical Treatment Negative comment? Perhaps it shouldn't receive a negative code at all. After all, what do patients know about the treatment they require?

Since we do not want to keep you hanging, here is how the PSMS qualitative coding scheme would be applied to these comments. First, we would code a Physician Positive for the "doctors . . . were terrific" phrase. We would do the same for the nurses mentioned in the same sentence. We do not consider this double-coding because the patient made specific attributions to doctors and nurses separately.

We would then code a Physician Negative for the "rude" medical resident. Since our decision rules specify medical students as being in years one through four of their four-year curriculum, the medical resident is coded as a physician. If the respondent had said, "the student doctor who was rude . . . ," then we would have coded this comment as a Medical Student Negative.

The echocardiogram issue would be coded a Doctor Negative because the attribution was specifically to the physician's clinical treatment. What's more, the negative code is assigned because it is the patient's perception that we are interested in measuring, not the medical and clinical appropriateness of the provider's decision. Had the patient stated, "I should have had an echocardiogram," we would have coded this as a Treatment Negative, since the physician was not specified in the comment.

As a last step in the process, the complete comment would be included in the data base for each coding decision so that the context of the comment would not be lost.

This example is not meant to bore you; it is intended to show you how hard it is to conduct accurate qualitative coding. The key is in how well you define your categories and the coding decision rules you create.

Your qualitative coding scheme should have its own quality assurance program

In qualitative coding it is extremely easy to introduce systematic bias. After all, not all coders will interpret the patient's written comments and coding decision rules in exactly the same way. Ideally, it would be wonderful to have at least three (or more) coders qualitatively code each survey. If there was less than total consensus on any coding decision, then the three coders could discuss how to resolve the disagreement. A coding supervisor could also be brought in to help resolve the issue.

Unfortunately, although an excellent approach methodologically, three coders are not operationally or fiscally feasible in the land of no more Hill-Burton monies and the fading away of fee-for-service reimbursement. An acceptable, although imperfect, solution is to first extensively train coders in the coding process; then, the most experienced coder should verify all the assigned codes. When disagreements occur the coder and verifier can discuss why the difference exists and work out a solution. With the PSMS we have also instituted this rule: If you aren't absolutely sure what code to assign a given comment, talk to another coder, preferably a senior coder, about it.

We have also instituted two other quality assurance techniques. First, each month coders get feedback from the verifier on where they did well and where they made coding errors. Second, we run ongoing qualitative coding quality assurance meetings, where difficult coding issues are presented and discussed.

Iterations

Qualitative coding schemes are not developed overnight. It takes trial after trial to develop a sound scheme. "Trial after trial" doesn't mean coding 100 surveys, revising your scheme once, and then "going with it." "Trial after trial" can mean ten to fifteen developmental iterations. In our experience, it took PSMS two years, qualitatively coding 3,000+ surveys, and roughly ten revisions before we were comfortable with our approach to qualitative analysis. Even then, we still constantly find ways to improve our system. Just as in writing quantitative survey items, you do not want to reinvent the wheel when developing qualitative coding systems. If you find another coding scheme that works, then get permission to begin with it. You can then tailor it to suit your organization's unique requirements if needed.

An Example of a Qualitative Coding Scheme

We will sketch for you an outline of the PSMS coding scheme so you may get a better idea of what a reasonably well developed qualitative system looks like. Then, in the last section of this chapter, we will discuss how qualitative data can be analyzed.

Category coding: First level

PSMS relies on 12 major first-level categories. A sample of some of these categories and their conceptual definitions are provided below.

A = Admitting. "Admitting" includes comments regarding the admission process or admitting staff. "Process" refers to items such as time waited, room readiness, bed availability, prearranged admission, and hospital transfer through the emergency department. "People" refers to behavior or attitude comments (for example, Rude, Loud, Pleasant, Friendly) and level of staffing comments.

B = Billing. "Billing" refers to the billing process, office, and personnel.

D = Doctors. "Doctors" includes comments referring specifically to a doctor, or any attributions to a physician (including attending physicians, interns, and residents), and comments concerning the availability and time of the doctor for the patient and family, the quality of test explanations and results, the quality of the care given, answering questions of patient and family, keeping the patient informed, discharge planning and follow-up care, understanding and empathy for the patient's condition, communication issues with patient and family in understanding terminology, behavior or attitude (for example, Rude, Unfriendly, Kind), and the change of attending or house staff during hospitalization.

E = Environment. "Environment" refers to general or specific comments about the medical complex facilities, including items about parking; ease of access or finding one's way around; signs; cleanliness; security or safety; convenience of public areas: rest rooms, telephones, cafeteria, vending areas, lobbies; renovation; waiting areas for specific floors or services (for example, intensive care units, atrium, surgery); decor and atmosphere throughout;

housekeeping functions in public areas; noise levels in general; level of staffing; behavior or attitude of an employee encountered in these settings; and public information (for example, receptionist, telephone operator). Please note that this category excludes comments attributed to the patient's room.

F = Food. "Food" includes comments about the efficiency and effectiveness of the dietary service as well as other process comments, including ordering and delivery of what was ordered, preparation and presentation of food, temperature and taste of food, menu selection and variety of food offered, snack availability, timeliness of meal, quantity of food, and placement of food trays in room. Comments concerning dietary staff issues (attitude and behavior) as well as the level of staffing are also presented here.

H = Housekeeping. "Housekeeping" includes comments pertaining specifically to housekeeping—cleanliness of the hospital, including patients' rooms; frequency of cleaning; sanitation; housekeeping personnel; and availability of patient supplies (for example, towels, washcloths).

I = Ideas. "Ideas" includes any comments on how we can improve current services and quality of care and new ideas for service or products.

M = Miscellaneous. "Miscellaneous" should only be used if comments relating to the patient's level of satisfaction (or other comment) cannot be placed under another defined category or if attribution cannot be made.

N = Nursing. "Nursing" contains comments concerning the attentiveness, responsiveness, friendliness, and courteousness of nurses, as well as staffing levels and working conditions of nurses. Included are comments concerning answering questions and providing information; answering the call button promptly; bringing things or doing things for the patient when requested; level of competency or skills; help to the bathroom; help in walking; delivery of medication in a timely manner; tending to personal hygiene; family treatment (behavior and attitude); and enforcement of hospital policies (for example, visitation, smoking). Comments are specifically about nurses.

O = Other staff/services. "Other staff/services" includes comments made about specific service areas not covered in other sections of this report—for example, comments about transportation, lab technicians, x-ray, social workers, pharmacy, and emergency department (unless specific to admitting process). Comments address the attitudes and behaviors of staff, staffing levels, attentiveness to needs of patients, answering questions, explaining tests, competency or skill level, and delivery of the service in an efficient and effective manner.

R = Room. This category includes comments about the patient's room that are not attributable to the housekeeping department fall under "room," including roommates, bed, facilities/maintenance (for example, a broken light switch), the attitudes of facilities maintenance staff, decor and atmosphere of the room, and noise level and temperature of room.

T = Treatment/diagnosis. This category includes comments relating to the technical issues and clinical management of diagnosis and treatment courses fall under "treatment/diagnosis," including comments regarding surgery: pre- and postoperation status, anesthesia, complication; responsiveness to special needs of special patient populations (for example, diabetics, transplants); unexpected or expected outcomes; timely acquisition of apparatus and medications; need for treatment and therapy; treatments done or not done (for example, radiation, respiratory, physical therapy treatments); too many or too few tests; allergic reaction or known allergies; medication prescribed and not given, or wrong medicine given; and IV maintenance and replacement.

Category coding: Second level

PSMS uses the direction of the respondent's value judgment or reaction as the basis for its second-level categorization. Comments within each first-level category are further broken down into Positive Comments, Negative Comments (critical), and Neutral Comments subcategories.

Category coding: Third level

Third-level analysis is conducted, though not in as systematic a manner. Instead of having predetermined third-level categories, we review all the positive and negative comments within each first-level category and assess if trends emerge. Themes within each second-level category that do emerge from quarter to quarter are then summarized statistically. For instance, we might note that 32 percent (of the Negative Admitting comments) concerned patients being upset with how long it took them to get to their rooms and 16 percent (of the Negative Admitting comments) concerned how difficult it was to read or complete the preadmission forms. But in a subsequent quarter, different third-level analysis trends may emerge. For instance, using the same example just cited, we might note in the following quarter that

29 percent of the Negative Admitting comments focused on respondents not being able to find the admitting area, which may not have been mentioned in the preceding month.

Theoretical basis—Attributional analysis

The PSMS relies on what we call *attributional coding*, the identification of the stimuli patients are referring to in their value judgment or reaction. Stated differently, attributional coding asks the question "To whom or to what does the patient attribute this value judgment, reaction, or stimulus?"

Each first-level category (listed above) in the PSMS qualitative coding system is designed around a large congruent attributional topic. For instance, if the patient says, "Nurse Jones responded to my requests for help very quickly, which I appreciated," it would be categorized as a Nursing Positive comment, since the patient attributed the comment to the nurse's behavior or action (stimulus). If the patient says, "All staff were great," it would be coded into (attributed to) our Miscellaneous Positive category because the stimulus—staff behavior or attitudes—is nonspecific. A major advantage to attributional coding is that it allows the manager to target where a strength or weakness in the organization may exist.

Decision rules and code books

The heart of sound qualitative analysis is the quality of the decision rules. As noted earlier, the decision rules give you the parameters you need to accurately interpret your data. Moreover, they serve to increase measurement reliability because they encourage formation of standardized coding protocols for a given coder and across different coders. A sample page from the PSMS qualitative code book is presented in Exhibit 9.1.

Unit of analysis

Level of analysis refers to coding categories and subcategories. *Unit of analysis*, as discussed in previous chapters, refers to how the data are broken down (analytically disaggregated) within the health care setting itself—for example, by nursing discharge unit or medical service. The utility of patients' written comments increases if we can aggregate their comments by nursing discharge unit, medical service, DRG, and physician identification number. You already know how this can be accomplished—the encoded label with complete information from the discharged patient's medical record—and the problems that can emerge when using encoded labels.

Exhibit 9.1   Sample Coding Rules from a PSMS Qualitative
Code Book Page

---

1. Multiple Comments

   If they all pertain to exactly the same topic, then group them together and code only once:

   F   "The meals were not very tasty—too much salt!"

   However:

   H   "The room was never cleaned (and it was too cold)."

   R   "(The room was never cleaned) and it was too cold."

2. Attribution

   Because we are measuring patient perceptions and expectations, when the patient attributes blame to a certain area or person, then the comment is coded accordingly:

   N   "Medication does not get dispensed properly when nurses are understaffed."

   But:

   T   "My medication was not properly dispensed."

   N   "My room was too noisy because the nurses were talking too loudly at the nurses station."

   E   "My room was too noisy because of the noise in the hall."

   R   "My room was too noisy—the vent in the room was terribly loud."

Relational data bases

Picture two data bases. The first is the quantitative data base, comprised of all of the numerical values patients circled or checked on the survey and all the information from the encoded label—for example, age, sex, DRG, nursing discharge unit, and discharge date. Importantly, the patient's survey (or case) identification number and discharge date are included in each line of quantitative data. A few lines from a quantitative data base might look like Exhibit 9.2.

The second data base is the qualitative data base, comprised of all the patients' written comments coded through the two levels of analysis described above. In addition, the patient's survey (or case) identification number and discharge date are included with each coded comment. A few lines of data from the qualitative data base might look like Exhibit 9.3.

In the parlance of today's "management information systemese," these two data bases are set up by the PSMS as *relational data bases*—they logically relate to one another because case identification number 202 in the

Exhibit 9.2   A Quantitative Data Base: A Partial Sample

		Label Data		
Case ID	Data from the Survey	Nursing Discharge Unit	Discharge Date (Month/Day/Year)	Other Encoded Label Data
201	3450914534232342345334234	3E	031291	31376875565124141234
202	3451002234555433234542113	2N	032191	24343493743299942344
203	3222344432345553422322333	3E	022891	21234985495845843285
516	3345553312111232111123332	2N	031491	34342997972346273463

Exhibit 9.3   A Qualitative Data Base: A Partial Sample

Case ID	First-Level Code	Second-Level Code	Actual Comment	Discharge Date (Month/Day/Year)
201	D(octor)	+	The doctor was the nicest person I ever met in my life.	031291
201	R(oom)	−	Why can't they supply hot water in the rooms?	031291
202	T(reatment)	+	The way they explained the chemotherapy to me took all my fear away. Thank you!	031291
203	Missing—no qualitative comments on this case			022891
516	E(nvironment)	+	I never heard any noise outside my room for six days. I appreciated this peace and quiet, given how sick I felt.	031491

quantitative data base is the same patient as case identification number 202 in the qualitative data base. Moreover, there is information contained in each data base that is useful in the analysis of the other.

Perhaps the most important example of their interrelationship is that the data from the encoded label—age, sex, medical service—in the quantitative data base are critical to better analyzing and understanding the written comments contained in the qualitative data base. If we could link the two data bases, we could look at, for example, all the Nursing Positive and Nursing Negative comments (qualitative data base) broken down by nursing discharge unit (quantitative data base). Or we could ask the computer and data base software to select all the cases where patients scored below 3.00 (five-point scale) on the overall nursing satisfaction indicator score from the quantitative data base, and print out each person's positive and negative nursing comments from the qualitative data base, further broken down by nursing discharge unit from the quantitative data base. Linking increases the power of patient satisfaction measurement enormously!

The question remains, How do we link the two data bases? The answer lies in another management information systems concept called the *indexing variable*. The indexing variable is the bridge that joins the two data bases. Within the PSMS the indexing variable is really two variables—the patient's medical record number and the patient's date of discharge. The medical record number is purposely not used alone as the indexing variable because the dates of different visits by the same patient would be confounding. Hence, we would be unable to distinguish one stay from another. Figure 9.2 graphically displays the relational data bases used by the PSMS.

Think of all the excellent research and operational questions you could ask—and perhaps find the answer to—through the use of these two relational data bases. Here are some examples:

- Physician ID number 452 shows the lowest overall physician satisfaction indicator score in our sample. I wonder what his or her

Figure 9.2   Relational Data Bases

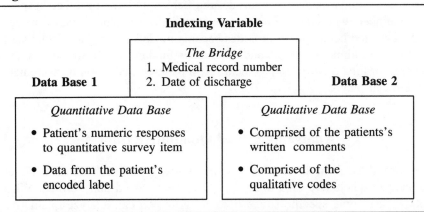

patients' written comments look like in general (all qualitative comments), particularly those specific to physician satisfaction (Physician Positive and Physician Negative comments)?

- Do written comments from oncology service patients differ from one another based on the patient's age?
- Do patients with overall satisfaction-with-stay scores below 5.00 (on a ten-point scale) make more negative comments about nursing, physicians, or their rooms?
- Do patients who strongly disagree or disagree that they will return to Health Hospital comment more negatively about the environment or their rooms?

The possibilities for important questions you now have some chance at answering are endless. As a result, the power of the patient satisfaction measurement tool grows even more.

Notable persons

What about all the names of hospital or outpatient staff that patients cite as doing a terrific job? How should these be managed? The answer is, through the qualitative data base. In the qualitative data base the names of staff cited by patients for excellence are entered, accompanied by the specific comments that patients make. This list is then compiled separately and generated for managerial use and distribution. Table 9.1 is an example of a "notable persons list."

It is important to again note that the staff person's name should be linked to the actual comment the patient makes about this person. This is psychologically more powerful than simply listing the staff person's name without the associated comment. Among the "notable persons," this should serve to reinforce and perpetuate desired behaviors. Among other hospital staff members who read the notable persons list, the notable persons' names and their cited behaviors or attitudes become models to emulate. Tying staff names to desirable behaviors and attitudes is fundamental to the service excellence or total quality management role a patient satisfaction measurement system can play.

Analyzing Coded Qualitative Data

It is very difficult to develop a sound qualitative coding scheme. It is easier to analyze qualitative data once they have been coded and verified. What follows are some specific suggestions on how you can analyze qualitative

Table 9.1   Notable Persons List, Health Hospital, June 1993

Case ID	Nursing Discharge Unit	Patient's Medical Service	Staff Name	Hospital Area/Position	Comment
345	3E	Oncology	Paula R.	Housekeeping	Her smile kept my spirits up during my stay.
389	2W	Medicine	Karol Henseler	MD	She always made time to answer my questions. She never was rushed with me.
421	4E	Pediatrics	Sandra Stranne	Nurse	What a profes-sional!
567	2W	Medicine	X, Susan*	Nurse	She cared about me and my con-cerned family, too.

*Often patients do not know or provide the "notable person's" full name. When this occurs, the partial name is entered along with any other identifying information. The hope is that knowing which medical service or nursing unit the patient was on will facilitate identification. When an *X* appears, as in Case ID 567, this indicates that the staff person's last name was not provided by the respondent.

data. Some important weaknesses and problems in analyzing qualitative data are also listed.

Read All Comments First

Before conducting any kind of analysis, we have found it useful to read through all of the qualitative remarks. At the risk of sounding too "soft," reading all of the comments allows us to get a feel for what our patients have to say.

Summarize Qualitative Data with Counts Analysis

Basic summaries

We strongly recommend that you conduct what we call *counts analysis*. Within each first-level category we count the number of second-level responses by category—positive, neutral, and negative comments, allowing us to develop percentages of positive and negative comments, which help health care managers to better conceptualize the data. For example, for "admitting" (July 1994) we might have 34 Positive Comments, 56 Negative Comments, and 10 Neutral Comments (34 percent Positive, 56 percent Negative, 10 percent Neutral). Of course, the Neutral category could be dropped, and a different set of percentages could be derived reflecting the ratio of positive to negative comments. In effect, this ratio would become an index that could be monitored longitudinally.

Third-level categorical summaries can be conducted as well. Using the above example, we might note that of the 56 positive comments, 37 were about excessive waiting times, 17 were about rude and insensitive staff, and 2 addressed other issues.

More complex summaries

Naturally, the encoded label could be brought into counts analysis via the relational data base methodology described above. For instance, we could look at all the coded nursing comments, break them down by nursing discharge unit, and generate a summary like Exhibit 9.4.

More complex summaries relying on the relational data base need not be limited to only nursing. Physician comments broken down by individual physician identification number could provide some very interesting information. Or the demographic and clinical information we have collected on our respondents could be used as breakdown variables as well. For instance, we could categorize all nursing comments by specified DRG or by patient age.

Trend Count Analysis over Time

Longitudinal analysis is critical to the efficacy of any patient satisfaction measurement system. Qualitative analysis lends itself to time trending in the same way that quantitative analysis does.

For example, one could trend the percentage of positive comments to total comments about dietary (and other first-level categories) over an eight-quarter period as shown in Figure 9.3.

Conduct word searches to answer operational and research questions

Today's data base management systems can do some extraordinary things. For instance, they can search through large volumes of text (qualitatively coded comments) for key words and phrases. How might this work?

Exhibit 9.4 Counts Analysis with Relational Data Base

---

5 South—Nursing Discharge Unit

   38 (76%) Positive Comments

   Seventeen of the positive comments had to do with the responsiveness of the nurses to the patients' requests.

   7 (14%) Negative Comments

   All negative comments had to do with what the patient perceived to be short-staffing problems. In three instances, it was the nurse mentioning this to the patient.

   5 (10%) Neutral Comments

5 North—Nursing Discharge Unit

   21 (64%) Positive Comments

   Twelve of these comments focused on how well the nurses helped the patients manage their fear and anxieties.

   10 (30%) Negative Comments

   Eight had to do with slow response time to patient requests.

   Two had to do with one nurse who was cited as being curt and abrasive.

   2 (6%) Neutral Comments

Suppose we are interested in studying the number of times patients indicated that housekeeping staff was impolite, discourteous, inconsiderate, rude, abrupt, or curt. These six words are our key words. We can now ask the computer (figuratively, of course), "Please look over all the qualitative comments for the last calendar year. Then, select out those negative comments about housekeeping (H−) where the words *impolite, discourteous, inconsiderate, rude, abrupt, and curt* appeared. Then, sort these by nursing discharge unit so I can tell what floors in the hospital these comments are coming from." The health care manager can, of course, ask—and perhaps answer—even more complex questions than these.

Weaknesses and risks

An unbalanced representation. A problem with the qualitative analytic approach just described is the presence of unequal representation in the data base; that is, patient number 201 may have five qualitative comments coded

Figure 9.3   An Example of Time Trending Qualitative Comments

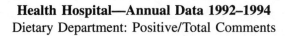

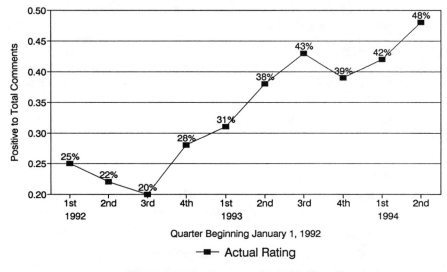

and entered into the data base, while patient number 354 may offer no comments. Unequal representation creates a potentially serious problem with the application of statistical procedures, longitudinal trending, and the generalizability of the qualitative data to the whole patient population you are serving.

The message, therefore, is threefold. First, if you intend to use any statistical procedures with your data, then make certain you get the assistance of a trained statistician. Second, be sensitive to bias in the data because a given patient may have generated a disproportionate number of written comments. Third, be careful about how you generalize the data from your sample of qualitative respondents. Any steps you can take to establish the clinical and demographic profiles of your qualitative respondents would be helpful in establishing generalizability. As noted in the preceding chapter, the qualitative analysis of initial nonrespondents' written comments would help you better understand the representativeness of your data as well.

Biases in your data. A major problem with qualitative analysis is that your coding decision rules can introduce bias into how the data are analyzed and interpreted. Health care managers who rely on their qualitative data must understand what these coding rules are and the types of bias they might introduce. Every time these data are reported, the researcher should make clear, in writing, what the limitations (for example, bias) to the data are.

Small sample sizes. Much of the analysis you will do with qualitative data deals with the percentage with which certain types of comments are made. A problem can result if the denominator used in calculating these percentages is smaller than, say, 30 comments. For instance, suppose there are only four medical student comments in a given reporting period, and we report that two (50 percent) of them were positive—this means very little, given the total number of medical student comments received. Moreover, the 50 percent value reported alone would be deceiving. It is a good idea to report both percentages and also the sample sizes that comprise them.

Subjectivity. Qualitative coding and analysis is by far the most difficult analysis to do properly because of the inherent biases and subjectivity built into the process. Coders are likely to disagree on how coding decision rules are applied. Patient comments will not always neatly fit into first-, second-, or third-level categories. Coder and researcher judgment flourishes in this process. These facts make it even more important that (1) you spend time standardizing your qualitative system, (2) you devote time and energy to coding quality assurance and staff training, and (3) you evaluate what you are doing on an ongoing basis. Subjectivity will always be a part of most qualitative coding schemes. Your goal should be to minimize it as much as possible.

Conclusion

The types of analytical frameworks described in this chapter only capture the proverbial "tip of the iceberg." Obviously, more sophisticated statistical techniques than simply counts analysis and breakdown analysis can be applied; however, this should not be done without the help of a trained statistician.

The power of the qualitative tool, when used alone or in conjunction with the quantitative data base, is potentially enormous. Developing relational data bases for patient satisfaction measurement is still new, though it is an exciting and potentially fruitful idea. In the next chapter, we hope you will see just how potentially powerful relational data bases can be in positively influencing organizational behavior.

PART V

USING PATIENT SATISFACTION DATA
FOR IMPROVED PATIENT SERVICES

10

PUTTING PATIENT SATISFACTION MEASUREMENT DATA TO WORK

Measuring patient satisfaction is a useless exercise and waste of resources if management chooses to do nothing with the data collected. The hospital's or outpatient clinic's management will lose credibility if they survey patients but do little to solve the problems that are identified. What's more, this may be unethical because the survey process explicitly suggests that the organization's management will do something with the information collected. We do not intend to start this chapter on a negative note, but the point is worth repeating: If you are not going to do anything with the data you collect, then don't bother collecting.

This chapter addresses what health care managers can do with the data collected. In many ways, this chapter is the most important in the book because a patient satisfaction measurement system is no better than the way in which managers use their data. Although some of the ideas presented here were briefly summarized in Chapter 1, they will be discussed here in more detail. In addition, some new ideas on using your data will be introduced.

There is a single and major theme throughout this chapter that should not go unnoticed: We believe that health care managers should develop a vision of patient satisfaction as something more than simply measuring patient exposure to stimuli, value judgments, and reactions. Instead, patient satisfaction can be viewed, and ultimately used, as an effective organizational development, strategic planning, and total quality management tool that touches all hierarchical levels, functions, and subsystems in the organization.

Using Patient Satisfaction Information Positively

Patient satisfaction measurement is doomed to a sudden and tragic death if the information collected is seen by health care staff as being used primarily for punitive purposes. Suppose nursing unit 4 East comes in with a patient satisfaction performance below the goals it had established earlier in the year. What happens next? If the manager's response is to blow up and read the nursing unit manager the riot act, then defensiveness and ultimate rejection of the patient satisfaction system is likely to occur. If the manager works collaboratively with the unit manager in trying to uncover the causes for lower-than-expected performance, then a positive response is more likely. This positive attitude will grow if the manager and unit manager also spend time together figuring out how to solve the problems they have mutually identified.

Patient satisfaction measurement gives health care management a powerful tool, but they must use it with extreme caution. For the first time, the health care manager now has relatively solid information on one of the most important quality-of-care outcome indicators, and this can be heady stuff. When we tell managers that we can feed back satisfaction ratings of physician care by individual physician, the unabashed joy in some the health care managers' eyes is evident from miles away. It is exactly this response that must be kept in check. Information is power, and the temptation to flex one's muscles is great—and also potentially destructive.

With this in mind, managers must use patient satisfaction data primarily to

- Make people accountable for their own high-quality job performance—not solely to document poor performance.

- Help staff identify ways to improve their performance—not to point fingers and blame other staff for lower-than-desired patient satisfaction performance scores.

- Help staff identify what they are doing well and reward them for this—not to identify who can be left alone, untouched, unnoticed, and unrecognized because the staff are doing a good job.

- Help improve the quality of care rendered—not to simply clean up the messes so that minimally acceptable standards of performance can continue.

This is not to say that health care managers should tolerate poor patient satisfaction performance among staff—obviously, they should not. However, positive human resource management strategies must be employed before staff are punished for poor patient satisfaction performance. Otherwise, your patient satisfaction measurement system will be destined for failure.

Creating User-Friendly Presentation Formats

The packaging of reports will have an impact on whether managers use your patient satisfaction feedback. Although there are clearly individual differences in what managers like and do not like, here are some general guidelines on how to design your feedback reports to maximize the chances that managers will read them.

Use Graphs and Numerical Tables

Data can be presented in three different forms: narrative text, tables of numbers, and graphs. Most managers prefer to see their data displayed graphically. After that, tables of numbers seem to be preferred. Narrative text that must be read appears to deter managers from using the data.

The PSMS project has experimented with many presentational formats in light of these preferences. We have had some success with the design in Exhibit 10.1.

This style of feedback corresponds to what we have found managers prefer. The graph is the dominant visual item on the page, followed by a table of numbers comprising the data for the graph. The narrative "observation" is concise and pointed in light of managers' general preference for less narrative text.

Avoid Presenting Too Much Information on a Page

Managers seem to prefer one or two concepts presented on each page of the report. We would rather give a manager a fourteen-page report that is not densely packed with information than one that is seven pages long and presents too much information on a single page.

Simplicity Encourages Use

Data presentation should be so crystal clear that managers can understand a page of feedback, including the graph, in less than 30 seconds. Thus, it is very important that graphs, in particular, are clearly labeled.

Provide a Glossary at the End of Each Report

The language (for example, mean, median) used in these reports can be confusing to many health care managers. Moreover, as management turns over and new people arrive, the language used in these reports could be confusing

Exhibit 10.1   A User-Friendly Presentation Format

Was the Waiting Time Acceptable?
Non–Emergency Room Admissions Only

Five-point scale (1 = Strongly Disagree; 5 = Strongly Agree)

Month	*Average Score*	*Standard Deviation*
June 1993	4.32	.89
July 1993	4.23	.91
August 1993	3.75	1.04
September 1993	3.72	1.07
October 1993	3.17	1.11

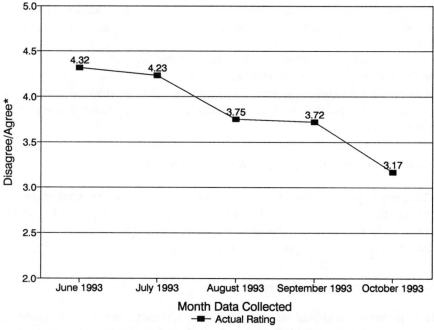

Month Data Collected
—■— Actual Rating

Note: Data apply to non-emergency room admissions only.
*1 = strongly disagree; 5 = strongly agree.

Observation

There has been a *consistent drop* in overall patient satisfaction with waiting time among non–emergency room admissions over the past five months.

to the newcomers as well. A glossary at the end of each report can help solve this problem.

Provide a Table of Contents and an Executive Summary

A table of contents will permit each manager to go directly to that section of the report that most interests him or her. We all know the frustration of flipping through pages of a report searching for the information we are most interested in and not being able to find it. A table of contents may solve this problem and also create an incentive to use the report.

A one-page executive summary should precede all reports. As you might expect, the summary should focus on highlights, such as major changes in the data over time or significant new findings.

Organize Data Logically and Consistently

In quantitative reports, it makes sense to organize the feedback around different sections of the survey—Preadmissions, Admissions, Food, Nursing Care, and so on. Within each major section, overall summary data should be presented first, followed by the more detailed by-item and breakdown analysis data. This is consistent with our recommendations on the sequencing of data analysis in Chapter 8.

To minimize relearning, report formats should remain standard from month to month or quarter to quarter. There should be a section at the end of each report called "New" or "Special Analyses." This will give you some flexibility with formatting, which you will undoubtedly need.

Present Qualitative Data as a Whole or in Subsets

Suppose you choose (as we do), to organize your qualitative reports in the following way:

Part I: How to use this report (one page in length)
Part II: Limitations, cautions, and caveats
Part III: Executive summary (one page in length)
Part IV: Graphs displaying the number and percentage of positive and negative comments for the reporting period and over time (fifteen pages in length)
Part V: The notable persons list (fifteen pages in length)

Part VI: Specific patient comments broken down by first- and second-
level categories and then sorted within each category by nursing discharge unit and medical service (forty pages in length)

The sum of those pages yields a report that can be seventy pages long. The
length alone will be a major disincentive to using the data.

One solution with which we are currently experimenting is to create
two kinds of reports. The first is the full-blown report that senior managers
may be most interested in reviewing since they may have the most interest
in learning about what patients are saying about all aspects of their stay or
visit. The second is an abbreviated report that includes only those sections
of the report that a given manager might be interested in. For instance, the
director of admitting might receive only that portion of the qualitative report
that applies to his or her area. This will cut down substantially on the amount
of reading (and paper).

Leave It Up to the End Users—The Managers

The bottom line, however, is that each organization's managers must decide
for themselves how they want to receive the data. Since it is the managers
who will be using the patient satisfaction data, it should be the managers
who decide how they want the information packaged and presented. Meeting with managers and discussing this issue with them is desirable when
developing your reporting formats. You can facilitate the process by giving
them alternative report formats to select from. The format should be decided
on not by what the report writer likes, but by what the managers like. After
all, they are the ones who must translate the data into diagnosis and action.

Provide Support for In-House Staff

Support for the in-house staff who are responsible for running the program
may seem like a small point, but it's not. Patient satisfaction measurement
systems, when used properly, create additional work, though ideally positive work. In-house staff support will be needed for a variety of important
activities:

- Copying reports
- Disseminating reports to the appropriate in-house staff
- Training other staff to use the patient satisfaction measurement sys-
tem
- Responding to triaged surveys
- Coordinating with quality assurance

- Coordinating with medical and nursing staff
- Revising the system if necessary
- Evaluating the system on an ongoing basis
- Coordinating with outside consultants if they are responsible for your report generation and analysis
- Coordinating with the management information systems staff for work relating to the encoded label
- Working with marketing and human resources management on how to use the data

Patient satisfaction measurement systems are run best out of one of three organizational areas:

1. Human resources departments
2. Marketing and planning departments
3. Departments of service excellence
4. Departments of patient relations

The in-house staff person in charge of the system will need to be given both time and some administrative support staff and training to use the system effectively.

Training Health Care Staff to Use Patient Satisfaction Measurement Data

It is naive to believe that all one has to do is deposit a ten-page patient satisfaction report on the manager's desk and he or she will take care of the rest. Yes, for some managers that is all you will need to do; for many others, though, a bridge needs to be built to connect the report to the manager's mind and ultimately to better decision making and action planning.

The foundation of this bridge is first to train managers in how their organization's patient satisfaction system works. One hour of training on the following topics may be all that is necessary:

- Why measuring patient satisfaction matters
- The costs and risks involved, and how these can be managed
- The positive philosophy of patient satisfaction measurement
- What the survey will look like
- What quantitative and qualitative data are
- How the survey sample is drawn

- How often and in what format the feedback will be disseminated
- Limitations of the system

A second hour of training should be devoted to teaching managers how to read and interpret their reports. This is not to say that managers are not smart enough to do this on their own; however, it is very easy to misinterpret patient satisfaction data, and managers need to be protected from this pitfall. Moreover, the more familiar managers are with the system, the more likely they are to open the report and start reading. The key is to make the system and the feedback it generates user-friendly and "user-helpful." Topics to cover in the second hour of training would include

- Organization of the reports
- Reading report tables, figures, and graphs
- A review of basic descriptive statistics
- A review of the language of patient satisfaction measurement: for example, What is "qualitative" and "quantitative" data? What does patient-mix adjustment mean? What is an overall indicator score?
- Drawing accurate conclusions from the data
- Avoiding misinterpretation of data

A third hour of training should focus on how managers can translate their data into more successful management practices. Topics covered might include

- Expressing positive and negative feedback to department- and unit-level staff
- Developing goal-setting programs based on patient satisfaction data
- Developing performance standards
- Using the data to enhance unit and individual job performance
- Using the data in training and staff development
- Developing problem-solving action plans based on the patient satisfaction feedback
- Rewarding staff for excellent patient satisfaction performance

Lastly, those staff responsible for administering the system should present one or two patient satisfaction in-service training sessions a year for all staff. Here, staff can be retrained in how to use the system, as well as be updated on any changes that have occurred in it. In addition, staff can be updated on recent research findings that have been identified from the data.

We cannot stress enough the importance of training. Like many evalua-tion processes, most of the time, money, and energy is directed at developing excellent measurement systems and hardly any resources are directed at training people on how to use the data collected and developing positive management action plans from these data. State-of-the-art patient satisfac-tion measurement systems in the 1990s and beyond should focus more and more on information utilization.

Some Ways to Use Patient Satisfaction Data

Goal-Setting Programs

In the field of organizational behavior, goal setting is one of the most re-searched topics. The findings from literally dozens of studies demonstrate that goal setting can improve job performance as long as the goals that are established have the following characteristics (Locke and Latham 1984):

- The goals must be clearly stated and measurable. A goal such as "Do your best this year in sales" is not as effective as a goal that states, "Do your best by increasing your sales by 12 percent over last year."
- The goals need to be valued or accepted by those seeking to accom-plish them; that is, an employee who does not believe in the right to smoke cigarettes should not work for a cigarette manufacturer.
- The goals must be challenging but attainable. If they are too hard, then people will give up trying to reach them, perhaps entering a state of learned helplessness (Seligman 1975). If they are too easy, they become uninteresting and people lose their drive to accomplish them.
- People seeking the goals must receive knowledge of the results; that is, they must get feedback to see how well they are progressing toward the accomplishment of the goals.

Patient satisfaction measurement lends itself almost perfectly to the establishment of patient satisfaction performance goals. We recommend the following strategies in developing these for your hospital or outpatient clinic.

Patient satisfaction goal setting must be a part of the hospital's or clinic's overall strategic plan

Health care organizations in the last decade have made major strides in the development and implementation of sophisticated strategic and tactical plans. The establishment of patient satisfaction performance goals should be integral to this planning process. Patient satisfaction performance targets must be set, and specific action plans to attain these targets must be identified as well. Accountabilities for implementing these action plans must also be defined.

Patient satisfaction goals must be integrated with the strategic plan

When "management by objectives" was being implemented in the 1960s and 1970s, one of the major problems with its successful implementation was that nonintegrated goals were being established throughout the organization. Hence, different subsystems—and even different individuals—within the organization were working at cross-purposes.

The same could happen with the establishment of patient satisfaction goals. For instance, admitting might establish a goal of decreasing average waiting time for patients to get to their rooms by 30 percent in a given year. However, this could run into direct competition with housekeeping's goal of spending 20 percent more time thoroughly cleaning patient rooms after patients are discharged.

When patient satisfaction performance goals are established, other department managers and senior management should be brought into the process to make sure that the goals, and the actions necessary to attain them, are not in conflict.

Goal setting should follow both top-down and bottom-up pathways

Beginning with the strategic plan, senior health care management must develop overall organizational patient satisfaction performance goals (top-down). "Top-down" does not mean a unilateral decision-making approach. Clearly, input from all levels in the organization must occur before these targets are set. Subsequently, middle managers, first-line managers, and, where appropriate, product-line managers should develop unit-level patient satisfaction performance goals that are consistent with those established through the strategic plan and by senior management. Nonsupervisory staff must also be brought into the goal-setting process.

Goals should be jointly set

The expectation among health care staff is that they will be made a part of the decision-making process, of which goal setting is certainly a part. Hence, unilateral goal setting may engender more resentment than commitment. Moreover, joint goal setting should include nonmanagerial employees. As noted above, all health care personnel should, in some way, be involved in the process.

Goal performance should be reviewed on an ongoing basis

All health care staff should receive ongoing feedback on their patient satisfaction performance for their own units and for the overall health care organization as well. Feedback can be disseminated through reports, team meetings, and the like.

Opportunities for goal adjustment should be made

One of the problems with "management by objectives" was that it became what Wendell French, author of many books on personnel management, called "rule by objectives." The established goals should not become rigid and unbending targets that cannot be adjusted. Unexpected contingencies can and will arise that require adjustment over time. Patient loads can increase, and sicker patients may be admitted at a higher than usual rate. This is not to suggest that goals should be adjusted on a daily basis. However, flexibility should precede rigidity.

Focus on goal progress as much as on goal attainment

Although goal attainment matters, improvement over previously established targets may be more important. Certainly, this focus is consistent with the positive philosophy of patient satisfaction that we discussed earlier in this chapter and in Chapters 1 and 2. In addition, it is consistent with contemporary thinking on total quality management and continuous quality improvement.

Goal performance should be shared to generate cooperation, not competition

It would be a mistake to sit down with the nurse manager from nursing unit 2 North and show the inpatient satisfaction results of their unit compared to those of all the other individual nursing units. Such a comparison would create the perfect medium for unhealthy intraorganizational competition. Showing this manager how 2 North compared to all other nursing units combined would be a better strategy, though some competition could still be fostered. The best strategy would be to show this manager the unit's patient satisfaction performance longitudinally—for example, over the last four quarters. As we have said all along, the best comparison to make is to yourself over time. A corollary to this is that the best person (unit) to compete with is yourself (your own unit) over time. The objective becomes improvement, and not winning at someone else's expense.

The organizational behavior literature suggests that goal setting works because it focuses employees' attention, helps them prioritize their activities, and requires them to think strategically. The opportunity to use patient satisfaction measurement in this way should not be lost!

Employee Performance Beyond Goal Setting

Beyond goal setting, there are other ways in which patient satisfaction measurement can positively influence job performance. Progressive hospitals, such as the Evanston Hospital, Glenbrook Hospital, and the Ohio State University Hospitals, are exploring ways to integrate patient satisfaction measurement into their employee performance appraisal system. This integration is an excellent use of the tool for the following reasons.

1. It increases the legitimacy of patient satisfaction measurement within the organization.
2. It increases employee accountability for delivering high levels of patient satisfaction performance (see below and in Chapter 2).
3. It offers managers a new way to reward health care employees based on objective criteria.
4. It offers an alternative to (not replacement of) supervisory perceptions of job performance.
5. It expands the breadth of performance criteria on which managers can rely.
6. It directs health care staff—both clinical and nonclinical—to think more about their patients.

Short of performance appraisals, the mere fact that health care staff know they are being evaluated may help to improve individual performance levels. The catalyst, as you already know, is the explicit performance accountability that patient satisfaction evaluation creates.

The "notable persons list" (described in Chapter 9) gives managers an opportunity to develop an informal role-model system within the organization. Listing staff persons' names, along with the desirable attitudes and behaviors they display, navigates employees in the direction of positive role models. Moreover, the need for recognition by patients may become contagious. In one PSMS site, the first time the notable persons list was circulated, staff who did not get cited by patients for excellent performance called the patient relations office to find out how they could get on the list!

At a time when health care managers are looking for ways to enhance job performance, patient satisfaction measurement offers one eminently feasible method.

Service Recovery: The Telephone Follow-Up Quality Communication System

Patient satisfaction data can be used to improve relations with patients the health care organization has disenchanted. By telephoning patients who have expressed dissatisfaction with their stay, it may be possible to reverse their negative attitudes. Here is how this can work.

The data base

At the PSMS sites, patients with overall satisfaction scores below a specified value are identified from the data base, including the patient's name, survey (case) number, and discharge date. Their actual survey is then pulled from our archives.

The telephone

These names and their corresponding surveys are then given to managers. Their job is to call the disgruntled patients and ask if there is anything the hospital (or clinic) can do to rectify the problem they cited on the survey. Approximately five to six patient names are given to each manager to contact in a given month. An effort is made to minimize the number of calls each manager must make so that this task does not become onerous.

At Ohio State University Hospitals, managers may receive surveys from patients who were dissatisfied with an area of the hospital that the managers are not responsible for. A nurse manager will get billing concerns and a billing manager will get clinical treatment concerns. Such a distribution is purposeful—for reasons discussed later in this section. It also can be risky—for reasons discussed later as well.

The training

Participating managers are put through a two-hour training program on how to effectively interact with patients during their follow-up telephone calls. Topics covered include

- Rules of confidentiality
- Listening skills and empathy training

- Avoiding becoming angry and defensive
- What the manager may and may not promise
- The emotional side of dealing with unhappy patients
- What to do after the telephone call is completed

Thus far, we have run 40 managers through the program at Ohio State University Hospitals. They have telephoned about 200 dissatisfied patients. Our evaluation of the program at this point in time is purely anecdotal, based on two debriefing sessions with the managers after they completed their calls. The second of these was videotaped for subsequent review.

In general we were astonished by the responses of both the patients and the managers who telephoned them. Here's what we found:

On the positive side, we heard telephoned patients say that they could not believe someone from the hospital either took the time to read their survey, bothered to call, or bothered to follow up on their concerns. This alone seemed to offset much of the bad will the hospital had engendered.

Many patients appreciated the opportunity to "just talk" to someone from the hospital about their experience. Even when calls were three months postdischarge, some patients still wanted to talk about their experience. Many patients simply appreciated the opportunity to verbally express their feelings.

Some patients attitudes about the hospital may have changed from either negative to neutral or negative to positive, as evidenced by comments like "I wasn't going to go back to your hospital, but after this call I think I will reconsider," or reports by some managers that the patient's hostility toward the hospital seemed to wane over time. The extent to which attitude changes occurred was not empirically determined. In addition, verbal statements about attitude change and softening voice tones are not necessarily predictive of whether or not the patient's attitude has actually changed and whether the patient will now recommend the hospital or return to it for future health care needs.

Positive benefits for the managers occurred as well. Many managers indicated that the telephone calls brought them closer to patients and helped them to better understand the problems patients face. To a business manager or management information systems supervisor, this can be an incredibly worthwhile experience because in many administrative areas it is easy to become psychologically and physically distanced from the patient. Our own assessment was that the managers' feelings of organizational commitment and job involvement also increased.

Another benefit was that managers were forced to learn about what happens in hospital areas other than their own, an excellent antidote to the age-old administrative problem of departmental myopia—only seeing workplace issues from your own or your unit's or your department's perspective.

At the risk of sounding corny, perhaps the best benefit for the managers was that it made them feel good about themselves. They were doing something they believed was worthwhile. It also embarrassed them to hear about some of the negative experiences for which their hospital may have been responsible.

What were the costs? From the patient's perspective the costs did not seem very high. Clearly, some patients may have felt intruded on or unwilling to relive their dissatisfying experience. We had no reported instances of patients hanging up, rudeness, or complaints to the hospital about the telephone call. However, some patients may still have felt unhappy about the call.

From the manager's perspective, the costs were different. Clearly, making the calls was time consuming. Some managers reported calls up to 45 minutes in length, though this seemed to be the exception rather than the rule. In addition, the program places an extra burden on the patient relations department if post–telephone follow-up action is needed.

Some managers found the experience a little depressing or disheartening because they were calling only dissatisfied patients. They indicated that they would like to call some satisfied patients as well, and this change will be introduced into the program. Some managers in our first group indicated that they wished they had been better psychologically "vaccinated" in the training session against the disheartening effects of dealing with only unhappy patients.

Problems have surfaced because managers in one functional area do not like managers from another area calling patients who have concerns with the former manager's staff or service (for example, a pharmacist calling a patient with a nursing complaint). If this concern arises it may be best to simply have nurses deal with nursing complaints, billing staff deal with billing complaints, and so forth. Although the integrative objective alluded to above is lost, there seems little sense in cajoling staff to behave in ways in which they are uncomfortable. Perhaps as the telephone follow-up programs become more ingrained within the organizational culture the cross-functional approach can be reconsidered.

Obviously, our evaluation of the efficacy of the program is nonsystematic and as methodologically full of holes as Swiss cheese. More work and research need to be done to evaluate the efficacy of this approach. The early returns are generally positive, although more so from the patient's perspective than the staff's perspective.

Quality of Care and Quality Assurance

Patient satisfaction data should be incorporated into the health care organization's quality-of-care/quality assurance programming. As argued throughout this book, patients are capable of making judgments about their clinical outcomes, clinical treatment, and the services rendered by the health care organization's staff. These data can be used to identify both strong and weak areas within the organization. Only naive health care managers believe that they already know what's going on in their organization. They may know what's going on from a manager's perspective, but not necessarily from a patient's perspective.

Some hospitals that we have worked with have already begun to use patient satisfaction data as part of their quality assurance monitoring system. Because of the encoded labeling system, hospitalwide and department/unit level patient satisfaction performance standards can be established and monitored. Patient satisfaction data can also be used for developing and monitoring patient satisfaction performance standards for nurses and physicians. As noted above, the quality assurance standards should be integrated into and congruent with the organization's overall strategic goal-setting process.

One of the best ways to use these data for quality-of-care purposes is to conduct research studies on the data you collect. For example, hospital management can investigate how patient satisfaction with physician and nursing care correlates with age, DRG, and acuity. These findings could have practical implications for patient treatment plans and patterns of patient care.

These data also can be used to bolster the health care organization's risk management program. Triaging of incoming surveys and the telephone follow-up quality communication program can be used to identify patients who may have an increased likelihood of taking legal action against the hospital or clinic. The triage system, in particular, can become part of risk management's "early warning detection system."

The quality-of-care and quality assurance implications of patient satisfaction measurement are only beginning to be realized. When they are fully thought out, we predict that a whole new set of ways to improve the well-being of our patients will be identified.

Other Research Uses

Patient satisfaction measurement offers health care managers a wonderful opportunity to evaluate the feasibility and efficacy of their own decisions and problem-solving interventions. Suppose nursing services are evaluating the efficacy of a hypothetical staffing pattern system for oncology services. The program is called "Stretch-a-Nurse." The idea is to develop RN/nursing aide dyads. Each RN is given a specific caseload. A single nursing aide is then assigned to only one RN as a staff assistant. The research question is, How does "Stretch-a-Nurse" affect the quality of care delivered? Patient satisfaction would be a part of the quality-of-care measure.

The presence of an ongoing patient satisfaction measurement system would allow for this natural field experiment to occur. The researcher can look at the patients' nursing satisfaction ratings among those patients affected by the "Stretch-a-Nurse" program and can compare these to the patients' nursing satisfaction ratings of those not affected. The key idea is that an ongoing patient satisfaction system allows health care managers to monitor the efficacy of many of the decisions they implement. In the above example, "Stretch-a-Nurse" can now be evaluated empirically through patient judgments in addition to the more traditional methods, such as debriefing nurses, nursing aides, and physicians on how well they felt the program went. The decision on whether or not to continue the program can now be based on more comprehensive and objective data.

Morale Building and Positive Organizational Building

A major challenge many health care managers face is how to maintain or improve employee morale at a time when the health care industry is asking more and more from each employee. Patient satisfaction data can be used for this purpose.

The notable persons list is a tremendous morale builder. It also reaffirms and makes perceptible many of the intrinsic reasons health care staff stay in the health care business. Staff have told us many times how satisfying it is to see their name on the list next to the positive comment the patient made.

Monitoring improvements in patient satisfaction performance can also boost morale. One hospital experienced significant improvement with overall patient satisfaction over a 16-month time period. Management sponsored an appreciation party for all the hospital staff to thank them for their efforts and successes.

In another instance, positive qualitative patient comments were enlarged and then printed on a large poster and hung in the hospital cafeteria. Every time employees went through the checkout line, they would see a large poster with a comment such as this: "If anyone in my family ever gets sick again, we'll come back to Health Hospital." A critical managerial issue here is to get staff to stop cognitively focusing so much on extrinsic rewards like pay raises and promotions and to get them to reidentify the intrinsic rewards their jobs offer (Deci 1971, 1975). The notable persons list represents intrinsic rewards—feedback from the work itself—of the highest level. The technical distinction between viewing patient positive feedback as an extrinsic or intrinsic reward gets blurred here. As used in this discussion, we are defining patient positive feedback as an intrinsic reward since the feedback is derived from the nature of the work itself—caring for the patient. Hence, when a nurse's action brings a smile to a discomforted patient's face, we would define this as an intrinsic reward.

The possibilities go on and on. In health care management we are very good at focusing on problems, weaknesses, and areas of concern. Employees often bemoan that they are told what they are doing wrong far more often than what they are doing right. Increased regulatory pressure has served to intensify the attention we all place on the negative—the proverbial "problem areas" or "areas of concern." To balance our focus some, patient satisfaction measurement can be used, liberally paraphrasing Blanchard and Johnson (1983), to "catch health care employees doing something right!" Using the data in this way should help to improve morale and the quality of the organization's climate.

Team Building

Getting health care staff to work as a team has been a growing concern among the health care managers we have worked with over the last five years. Patient satisfaction data can be used to facilitate this process. The reason goes back to our discussions on goal setting and employee job performance.

One of the most potent forces that can pull a team together or build team cohesiveness is commonly shared and valued goals. It is no news to anyone that superordinate goals can override the dysfunctional effects of petty group differences, dysfunctional group conflict, turf battles, and arguments over space and scheduling. Increasing patient satisfaction can be identified as a superordinate goal around which many health care staff can rally. Specifically, this superordinate goal can be used to develop team attitudes and behaviors since it is the need to help the patient that motivates so many health care staff to begin with. The patient satisfaction data collected can be used to establish team goals and monitor team progress toward them.

Effective teams are also successful at identifying a problem area, owning up to it when it is their responsibility, and finding and implementing workable solutions. Patient satisfaction data can be used to help teams work in this problem-solving way. What's more, these data can serve as a catalyst or focal point for total quality managment and quality circle programs, and other group-based performance-enhancing management approaches.

Two key cautionary notes are called for. First, team building is good as long as it does not foster competition between groups that must work interdependently. Second, the team goals that are centered around patient satisfaction issues must be consistent with those of the organization's strategic plan.

Training and Orientation Programs

Patient satisfaction data can be extensively used for in-services and orientation programs, as is currently being done in some PSMS sites. Qualitative data should be particularly useful here. Trainers and managers can use this data to identify examples of appropriate and inappropriate staff attitudes and behaviors. What should make them so useful is that they are real examples from real patients who really did stay or visit their hospital or outpatient clinic.

In orientation programs, taking the time to explain the patient satisfaction measurement system and sharing some recent findings should serve as the first step toward creating patient satisfaction awareness and accountability among new staff. Discussing patient satisfaction in the orientation program also sends a powerful message to new employees: This hospital cares what its patients think and feel.

External Marketing Uses

As noted in Chapter 1, there are many potential marketing applications for patient satisfaction data. Just having a system can help create, in the consumer's mind, the image of a health care organization that cares what its consumers think. Extracting patient testimonials (with their written permission) from the qualitative data set and including them in brochures and advertisements is an excellent use of this data. Advertising positive quantitative outcomes is a logical extension of this idea. In one PSMS site, actual summary data were used in an advertisement that showed how satisfied patients had been with a particular service.

External marketing implies more than only marketing to consumers. It also implies marketing for staff recruitment purposes. A track record of strong patient satisfaction performance could help in the recruitment of physicians, nurses, and other health care employees. What is more, the existence of a patient satisfaction measurement system sends the same message to prospective employees as it does to the consumer: This is an organization that values its patients.

Fund-Raising Purposes

The following scenario is a demonstration of one of the worst public relations nightmares.

The Scenario: The development office of Health Hospital decides to do a direct mail campaign for soliciting contributions from all patients who have been discharged from the hospital in the last year. The letters are mailed out to every single patient and patients begin to respond. A letter is received back to the attention of the development office with a copy to the president from Mr. Rick R. (Really) Mad, attorney-at-law. In his letter Mr. Mad states: "I cannot believe that Health Hospital has the unmitigated gall to send a letter requesting that I contribute annually to assist in supporting its activities! It is beyond my comprehension that you did not pay any attention to the fact that I not only threatened to sue you while in the hospital (due to the inappropriate removal of my gall bladder), but that you did not even bother to check with your legal offices to know that I have filed my intent to sue. I even spoke with your patient representative regarding this matter. Don't you people communicate with each other? This is just one more confirmation of my suspicion that your hospital does not know what it is doing!!! Do you honestly believe that I would give you one dime for anything? You know what you can do with your request!!!"

Common sense says to most of us that mass mailings for development efforts should never be done, but it still happens. It is not the most effective utilization of development budgets, nor is it a rewarding experience for your hospital when contact is made with a dissatisfied patient. Many Americans really do believe that it "takes a lot of gall" to ask for money when they have perceived a "wrong" by a hospital, or any other entity for that matter.

Patient satisfaction measurement systems can assist development efforts by sorting out the grateful and appreciative (satisfied) patients, who may be more likely to give or not be offended if solicited. On an overall satisfaction scale of one to ten ("one" being extremely dissatisfied and "ten" being extremely satisfied) with a hospital experience, a criterion of all patients who rated Health Hospital a "nine" or "ten" could be utilized for mailing. More sophisticated sorting methods might be applied as well. Sorting patients on the basis of zip code and age, for instance, can add precision to the development campaign. Triaging surveys for development purposes is another potential use.

Since many of the dissatisfied patients are also known to your patient relations staff, your risk manager, or both, it is always a good idea to check with them prior to approaching any patient for money. Much of their information concerning dissatisfied patients will also come from patient satisfaction surveys that have been previously triaged at receipt. Although sorting surveys in this way may not totally eliminate contact with a dissatisfied patient, it certainly will change the odds.

Of course, sorting can only be done, and a listing generated for development, with the patients who have returned patient satisfaction surveys. If Health Hospital's rate of return is about 35 percent, then at least 35 percent of the patients are being screened. Once again, the odds have changed and you have enhanced the likelihood of finding patients who really would like to give to your hospital.

There are serious ethical considerations to fund raising in this way that must be considered. First, if the health care organization is legally a for-profit entity, then this approach would be akin to IBM asking for donations, using sales receipts or warranty information to generate their solicitation lists.

Second, one must ask if it is ethical to use patient satisfaction survey data in this way. Patients may have thought that by responding to the survey they were trying to help improve services or reward excellent care. It may be a nasty surprise to learn otherwise. Therefore, if this methodology is going to be employed, we strongly suggest that you have an item on the survey that asks patients for permission to follow up with them for research, development, and other purposes. Your hospital's or outpatient clinic's legal counsel should review the issue as well.

Third, satisfied patients may be very resentful that the information they are providing is helping the hospital to obtain even more dollars than they already have been billed for. Hence, we run the serious risk of turning happy consumers into angry ones.

Clearly, using patient satisfaction surveys for development purposes can only be implemented after a great deal of soul searching, and legal and ethical counsel, and with a willingness to live with certain potential negative consequences.

There are two last issues to consider. First, some development efforts in hospitals have a tendency to concentrate on those individuals (your VIPs) who can give the largest contributions or endowments to the hospital. Their assumption is "more bang for the buck" in terms of their resources. There is a marketing and public relations value to recruiting and accepting the $25 from 60-year-old Mrs. Doe, who has a loyalty to your hospital and who will be spreading positive word of mouth. Mrs. Doe may give you only $25 a year for development, but what she will do for your hospital in new patients and overall community image could be worth far more.

Second, although much of what we have written is cautionary, let us not forget how much quality health care means to our well-being, as the following example illustrates:

When I rushed my son to the hospital they said he might not make it. The medical student had tears in his eyes as he relayed this to me. I couldn't believe this was happening to my family. I had heard about it, but it could never happen to us.

I had never seen doctors more worried in my life as they tried to get my child out of shock. I have never been so scared and have never seen medical professionals look so scared.

Fortunately, the staff's excellent care saved my child's life and he has now fully recovered. Two weeks postdischarge, we received a solicitation letter in the mail from the hospital asking us if we wanted to donate. My wife and I looked at each other and simultaneously said, "How much can we afford right now?"

Conclusion

This chapter has attempted to point out a number of ways patient satisfaction data can be used to benefit the organization, its patients, and its employees. Stated differently, it is a chapter that focuses on turning data into information, and information into positive managerial action.

The benefits of patient satisfaction measurement are comprehensive, and health care managers must understand this to maximize the utilization of these data. Perhaps even more important than this, health care managers must philosophically believe that the empirical evaluation of patient satisfaction is as important to their organization's success as is the budgetary analyses they conduct on an ongoing basis and the board relationships they work so diligently to build.

If close readers think they hear an editorial message here, they are right. We believe that health care managers have gotten too far away from their patients, and perhaps too close to health care finance, strategic planning, and other primarily administrative or managerial activities. We are not saying that these areas are not critical for managerial attention and organizational success—they are! But so is the patient, who unfortunately is too easily lost in the shuffle. A commitment to patient satisfaction measurement is one step in the direction of elevating our patients to the high priority they deserve.

EPILOGUE

If you were ever a student in a health care management class some 15 or 20 years ago, then chances are that you heard a professor once say, "Administrators (class), your real consumers are your physicians. This is the group you must satisfy!"

Today, if you were sitting in the same class and the instructor was not using parched and yellowed notes, you would hear a much longer and more comprehensive statement: "Managers (class), you have many consumers. Physicians are one group of consumers because they still represent a large portion of your input and production function. If you have no physicians, then you have no referrals or admissions. If you have no referrals or admissions, then you will have serious trouble generating revenue. Your board represents another group of consumers as well. In the 1990s and beyond, contemporary thinking in human resources management suggests that your employees need to be viewed and treated like consumers, too. And last, though not least, are your patients. They are consumers you must satisfy as well."

This book was written to help you better understand and ultimately work with your patient groups. However, when viewed from a systems perspective, the implications extend well beyond only patients. By helping patients you may increase your chances of also satisfying your other important consumer groups, as long as your patient satisfaction system actually does lead to more satisfied patients, higher-quality care, and better job performance. Physicians may be held less accountable by their patients for problems that are beyond their control. Perhaps, these problems will be stopped or solved before the doctor even hears about them. Board members may hear fewer complaints and face fewer lawsuits. More satisfied patients may also result in less staff burnout and stress. But these are all from the debit side of the ledger.

From the positive side, satisfied patients may be more likely to return to your organization, spread the good news of their high-quality care and services, and cope with the emotional turmoil of sickness. Maybe more satisfied patients experience better clinical outcomes.

This book does not identify specific tools and techniques for making patients more satisfied. Interventions like empathetic listening, improving patient communications, and protecting patient rights were purposely not discussed because the focus of this book is on diagnosis and general management action, not working one-on-one with dissatisfied patients. If we were successful in helping our readers to become better evaluators and diagnosticians, then better defined and targeted interventions to solve patient satisfaction problems should logically follow.

This book has another purpose, which we alluded to in the last chapter. Its purpose is to redirect some of our managerial attention on that which we are about—helping our patients. The study of health care finance, planning, and marketing is about a decade ahead of our knowledge base on patient satisfaction. For every dollar health care organizations have spent on developing practical cost-accounting systems (fiscal evaluation), we believe a penny or less has been spent on developing ways to assess what our patients think and feel about the care and services we render. If this ratio (100:1) is correct, then it seems to us that some balance needs to be restored.

Some of today's health care organizations can be likened to a garbled and blurred mosaic of fragmented activity. When one looks at these confused organizations one may wonder, "How does it all get done? How does the patient get cared for?" Health care managers are under enormous pressure to "clean it up," "keep costs reasonable," "maximize productivity," "maintain market share," and "fulfill significant social responsibilities." Perhaps, our patients are one important place to look to find some of the answers. This book, hopefully, will help all health care managers and practitioners to look more closely and accurately.

APPENDIX

WORKSHEET FOR COST OF LOST REVENUES FOR VARIOUS CONTINGENCIES

Direct Costs of Dissatisfied Patients

Total discharges	14,500	14,500	14,500	14,500	14,500	14,500	14,500
Patients who have choice	35.00%	35.00%	45.00%	45.00%	35.00%	35.00%	45.00%
Total discharges with choice	5,075	5,075	6,525	6,525	5,075	5,075	6,525
Percent who say, "never return"	2.48%	5.00%	2.48%	5.00%	2.48%	5.00%	5.00%
Number saying, "not returning"	125.86	253.75	161.82	326.25	125.86	253.75	326.25
Controllable dissatisfied	90.00%	90.00%	90.00%	90.00%	90.00%	90.00%	90.00%
Total not returning, controllables	113.274	228.375	145.638	293.625	113.274	228.375	293.625
Percent making good on threat	40.00%	40.00%	40.00%	40.00%	30.00%	30.00%	30.00%
Number actually not returning	45.310	91.350	58.255	117.450	33.982	68.513	88.088
Cost of lost patient revenue	$3,626.00	$3,626.00	$3,626.00	$3,626.00	$3,626.00	$3,626.00	$3,626.00
Subtotal A	$164,292.61	$331,235.10	$211,233.36	$425,873.70	$123,219.46	$248,426.33	$319,405.28

Word-of-Mouth Effects

Total number dissatisfied	125.86	253.75	161.82	326.25	125.86	253.75	326.25
Number of people they speak to	6	6	6	6	6	6	6
Total number bad-mouthed to	755.16	1,522.5	970.92	1,957.5	755.16	1,522.5	1,957.5
Percent who have a choice	35.00%	35.00%	45.00%	45.00%	35.00%	35.00%	45.00%
Total with choice bad-mouthed to	264.306	532.875	436.914	880.875	264.306	532.875	880.875
Percent bad-mouthed to going elsewhere	12.50%	12.50%	12.50%	12.50%	12.50%	12.50%	12.50%
Total going elsewhere	33.038	66.609	54.614	110.109	33.038	66.609	110.109
Lost revenue	$3,626.00	$3,626.00	$3,626.00	$3,626.00	$3,626.00	$3,626.00	$3,626.00
Subtotal B	$119,796.69	$241,525.59	$198,031.27	$399,256.9	$119,796.69	$241,525.59	$399,256.59

Totals

Subtotal A	$164,292.61	$331,235.10	$211,233.36	$425,873.70	$123,219.46	$248,426.33	$319,405.28
Subtotal B	$119,796.69	$241,525.59	$198,031.27	$399,256.59	$119,796.69	$241,525.59	$399,256.59
Total	$284,089.30	$572,760.69	$409,264.63	$825,130.29	$243,016.15	$489,951.92	$718,661.85

BIBLIOGRAPHY

Bem, D. J. "Self-Perception: An Alternative Interpretation of Cognitive Dissonance Phenomena." *Psychological Review* 74 (1967): 183–200.

Blanchard, K., and S. Johnson. *The One Minute Manager: The Quickest Way to Increase Your Own Prosperity.* New York: Berkley, 1983.

Campbell, D. T., and J. C. Stanley. *Experimental and Quasi-Experimental Designs for Research.* Chicago: Rand McNally, 1963.

Cunningham, L. Paper presented at the Conference on Quality Assurance. Washington, DC, 1987.

Deci, E. L. "The Effects of Externally Mediated Rewards on Intrinsic Motivation." *Journal of Personality and Social Psychology* 18 (1971): 105–15.

Deci, E. L. *Intrinsic Motivation: Research and Theory.* New York: Plenum, 1975.

Festinger, L. A Theory of Cognitive Dissonance. Stanford, CA: Stanford University Press, 1957.

Fishbein, M., and I. Ajzen. *Belief, Attitude, Intention, and Behavior: An Introduction to Theory and Research.* Reading, MA: Addison-Wesley Publishing, 1975.

Fiske, S. T., and S. E. Taylor. *Social Cognition.* New York: Random House, 1984.

Greenberger, D. B., and S. Strasser. "The Development and Application of a Model of Personal Control in Organizations." *Academy of Management Journal* 11 (1986): 164–77.

Healthcare Financial Management Association (HFMA). *The Hospital Industry Performance Report.* William O. Cleverly, project director. Columbus, OH: Ohio State University, Division of Hospital and Health Services Administration, 1989.

Locke, E., and G. Latham. *Goal Setting: A Motivational Technique That Works.* Englewood Cliffs, NJ: Prentice-Hall, 1984.

Meterko, M., E. Nelson, and H. R. Rubin. "Patient Judgments of Hospital Quality: Report of a Pilot Study." *Medical Care* 28, no. 9 (1990): S40.

Moser, C. A., and G. Kalton. *Survey Methods in Social Investigation*, 2d ed. New York: Basic Books, 1972.

Nelson, C. W., and J. Niederberger. "Patient Satisfaction Surveys: An Opportunity for Total Quality Improvement." *Hospital & Health Services Administration* 35, no. 3 (Fall 1990): 409–27.

Nisbett, R., and L. Ross. *Human Inference: Strategies and Shortcomings of Social Judgments.* Englewood Cliffs, NJ: Prentice-Hall, 1980.

Rosselli, V. R., J. M. Moss, and R. W. Luecke. "Improved Customer Service Boosts Bottom Line." *Healthcare Financial Management* (December 1989): 21–28.

Schneider, D. J., A. H. Hastrof, and P. C. Ellsworth. *Person Perception,* 2d ed. Reading, MA: Addison-Wesley Publishing, 1979.

Seligman, M. E. P. *Helplessness: On Depression, Development, and Death.* San Francisco: Freeman, 1975.

Singh, J. "Consumer Complaint Intentions and Behavior: Definitional and Taxonomical Issues." *Journal of Marketing* 52 (1988): 93–107.

Strasser, S. *The Patient Satisfaction Measurement System.* Columbus, OH: Ohio State University College of Medicine and University Hospitals, 1988.

Technical Assistance Review Programs (TARP). "Measuring the Grapevine— Consumer Response and Word of Mouth." Study Conducted for the Consumer Affairs Department of the Coca Cola Company by TARP, August 1983.

Yankelovich, Skelly, and White. *The Charitable Behavior of Americans.* Washington, DC: Independent Sector, 1986.

INDEX

Accountability, 18, 19, 176, 186
Attributional coding, 162
Average scores, 136–37

Blanchard, K., 192
Breakdown analysis: conceptual model for, 142; first level of, 143; multidimensional, 147; second level of, 144, 145, 146; third level of, 146–47

Clinical information, 69
Clinical outcomes: and patient perception, 100
Clinical treatment: quality of, 99–100
Coding: clarity, 156, 161–62; first-level categories, 155, 159–61; and health care management, 154; overlap in, 155; rules of, 158; second-level categories, 155, 161; staff for, 158; third-level categories, 155
Cognitive consistency, 82
Cognitive psychology, 53
Confidentiality: and encoding, 73; patient satisfaction data and, 41, 43–44
"Controllable dissatisfied," 6, 10
Counts analysis, 167–68, 169; time based, 168–71
Critical mass, 114
Cronbach alpha reliability statistic, 140
Cunningham, L., 17

Data analysis, 132–52, 162, 179; and accuracy of data, 132–33; breakdown analysis, 141–47; descriptive, 133–37; overall indicator scores, 137–41; patient-mix adjustment, 148–49; software for, 131–32; unit of, 162; verification, 132–33
Data base: qualitative, 163, 164, 165, 166; quantitative, 163, 164, 165; relational, 165, 168, 169
Data entry: coding, 130, 132; software for, 131; staff training, 130–31; verification, 130
DBASE IV, 131
Demerol, 41
Demographic information, 69
Doctor-patient relations, 52

Employee morale: and patient satisfaction measurement, 20–21
Employees: as consumer, 197; productivity, 3, 18–20, 182, 186
Encoded label, 101, 141, 146, 152, 162; and counts analysis, 168; data from, 165
Encoding, 70–71, 75; accuracy of, 73; advantages, 71–72; and confidentiality, 73; logic of, 69–73; problems with, 72–73; and return rate, 69, 72

Evanston Hospital Corporation, xiv, 18, 21, 186
External validity, 123
Extrinsic rewards, 191

Factor analysis, 140
False consensus bias, 93
FOXPRO, 131
French, Wendell, 185
Fund-raising: and patient satisfaction, 24, 121, 193–96

Glenbrook Hospital, 186
Goal setting: and patient satisfaction, 183–84; and progress, 185

Healthcare Financial Management Association, 5
Health care management: and patient satisfaction measurement, xii, 11, 37, 181–82
Health care organization: and patient satisfaction measurement, xii, xiii, 27
Hospital board: as consumer, 197

IBM, 195
Incentives: use of, 121
Indexing variable, 165
Intraorganizational competition, 185
Intrinsic rewards, 191

Jessee, William F., 39
Job performance: feedback, 22; and patient satisfaction data, 3, 19, 182, 186
Johnson, S., 192
Joint Commission on Accreditation of Healthcare Organizations, 39

KCA Research, 17

Lawsuits: causes of, 17
Lay evaluation, 36
Leniency effect, 85, 137
Logic check analysis, 132
Luecke, R. W., 5

Malpractice suits: and patient satisfaction measurement, 10, 36
"Management by objectives," 184, 185
Marketing: and patient satisfaction measurement, 3, 12–17, 113, 193
Mean, defined, 133
Median, defined, 133
Median scores, 136–37
Medical Care, 91
Meterko, M., 60, 68, 120, 125
Mode, defined, 133
Mortality rates, 21
Moser, C. A., 10
Moss, J. M., 5

Negative feedback, 64, 85
Nelson, C. W., 100
Niederberger, J., 100
Nonrespondents, 123–24; telephone survey of, 125
Nosocomial infection rates, 21
Notable persons list, 166, 167, 186, 191
Nursing staff: and patient satisfaction measurement, 38, 96

Ohio State University, 60, 63; College of Medicine, xiv, 91
Ohio State University Hospitals, xiv, 18, 21, 96, 186, 187, 188
Overall indicator scores: advantages, 139; risks, 139–41

Parkside Associates, 91
Patient: as consumer, 197; information about, 69–70
Patient acuity, 148
Patient-mix adjustment, 142, 148–49, 152, 182
Patient satisfaction: and billing, 140; definition of, 49–56; and doctor-patient relations, 52; dynamic model of, 60–61, 64; facets of, 56–60; and health care management, xii, 11, 37, 181–82; individual differences in, 53–56; and malpractice suits, 10; and market share, 11; moderators of, 61; and overall planning, 183–84; and

quality management, xii; and revenue loss, 6–12; and staff, 10, 11; as a tool, 175

Patient satisfaction data, 9–10, 45–46, 149; abuses of, 42–45; and accountability, 176; accuracy of, 152; back up of, 152; confidentiality of, 41, 43–44; and employee morale, 191–92; encoding of, 72; ethics of, 195; and fund-raising, 193–96; glossary for, 177; and goal setting, 183–86; and incentive use, 121; interpreting of, 41–42; and job performance, 3, 19, 182, 186; organization of, 179; ownership of, 43; and patient relations, 187; presentation of, 177, 178, 180; qualitative, 97; and quality assurance monitoring system, 190; and quality of care, 176, 189–90; and risk management, 190; summary of, 179; and team building, 192; and training, 192–93; use of, xii, xiv, 176, 181–96

Patient satisfaction measurement: and accountability, 186; bad data for, 45–46; benefits of, 3, 34–35, 42, 196; of clinical treatment, 100; costs of, xiii, 27–33, 46, 114–16; ethics of, 44; expectations, 33–35; feedback from, 20–21, 39; and fund-raising, 24, 121; and health care management, xii, 11, 37, 181–82; and health care professionals, 19; and job performance, 3, 19, 182, 186; legal questions about, 36, 45, 186; and marketing, 3, 12–17, 113; methods of, 40, 57–60, 63, 75, 121, 168; and nonpatient responses, 73–75; and nonrespondents, 124; norms, 32, 150; and overall satisfaction, 148, 149; problems of, xiii, 18; and problem solving, 190; and qualitative, 63–64, 109, 153; and quality of care, 3, 22–24; quantitative, 61–63; resistance to, 35–42; and revenues, 3–12; and risk management, 3, 17–18, 190; scores, 149–51; and staff, 3, 20–21,

32, 35–36, 38, 96, 180–81; subjects of, 44; time tracking, 151; unit of analysis, 30, 97; use of, 12, 20, 39, 40, 175; validity of, 123

Patient Satisfaction Measurement System Project, xiv, 5, 68, 69, 75, 88, 91, 107, 119, 130, 186, 193; code book of, 132, 134–35; and coding, 157–63; data, 74; and low satisfaction patients, 187; mailing label, 71; measurement methods, 63; presentation formats, 177; research for, 60

Patient testimonials, 193

Physicians: as consumer, 197; and patient satisfaction measurement, 35–36, 96

Positive response set bias, 137

Present value cost, 11

Press, Gainey Associates, 91

Productivity of employees, 3, 18–20, 182, 186

Program: validation of, 131–32

Psychological outcomes: and patient perception, 100

Qualitative analysis: categories, 154–59; coding, 153–66, 170; decision rules, 162; risks, 169–71; subjectivity, 170, 171; time, 168

Qualitative data, 30, 182; analysis of, 166–71; counts analysis, 167–68; and negative feedback, 64; presentation, 179–80; sample size, 171; statistical procedures with, 170

Qualitative questions, 96, 109; distribution, 109–10; and market research, 111–12; use for, 111

Quality assurance: and patient satisfaction, 21; protocols, 46

Quality assurance monitoring system: and patient satisfaction data, 190

Quality circle programs, 192

Quality management, xii, 192

Quality of care, 21–24; and patient satisfaction data, 176, 189–90

Quantitative data, 182

Quantitative methods, 61–63; and leniency effect, 85; response scales, 103

Quarterly sampling: and critical mass, 114–15; timing of, 115

Range, defined, 133
Range check analysis, 132
Report formats, 179
Respondents: nonpatient, 73–75; profile of, 123
Response scales: continuous, 103, 104; dichotomous, 104; midpoint of, 104
Return rates, 122; and incentives, 121
Revenue loss: and costs, 10
Risk management: patient satisfaction measurement, 3, 17–18, 190
Rosselli, V. R., 5, 10
"Rule by objectives," 185

St. Vincent Medical Center, xiv
SAS. *See* Statistical Analysis System
"Silent dissatisfied," 6
Social psychology, 53
SPSS. *See* Statistical Package for Social Sciences
Standard deviation, defined, 133
Statistical Analysis System (SAS), 131
Statistical Package for Social Sciences (SPSS), 131
Statistics: sample size, 142
Stimuli: and patient satisfaction, 50–51, 52; perception of, 53, 56; and value judgments, 64
Survey: billing satisfaction data for, 140; completeness of, 86–87; confidentiality of, 83–85, 86, 122; costs of, 88; cover letter for, 89, 90; data, entry of, 129–31; design of, 79–83, 87, 88, 91, 97, 122; follow-up for, 122, 187–89; frequency of, 113–16; front matter of, 83–88; instructions for, 89; legal review, 102; and marketing, 87; and nonrespondents, 123–24; nursing data for, 138; parking problem data for, 137; pedagogical tools in, 87; qualitative comments in, 82–83; quantitative questions in, 91–109; quarterly sampling, 114, 115; respondents of, 123; return rates of, 121; sample size, 115; testing, 102; waiting time data for, 136. *See also* Survey distribution; Survey population; Survey questions
Survey distribution: at discharge, 117–18; during stay, 116–17; and health care staff, 117; methods of, 118; timing of, 119–21
Survey population, 67–69; clinical composition, 68; demographic composition, 68
Survey questions, 81–82, 105; forced choice type, 107; information value of, 98; input for, 99, 102; and market research, 106; order of, 81; qualitative, 109–12; quantitative, 91–109; rank order type, 106–7; specificity of, 94; wording of, 92–93, 98–99

Technical Assistance Review Programs, 5
Telephone follow-up: and attitude changes, 188; costs, 189; training program, 187
Telephone surveying, xv
Triage, 17–18, 28, 31

"Uncontrollable dissatisfied," 6, 10
Unplanned readmissions, 21
Upper Valley Medical Center, xiv

Value judgments, 51, 52, 64

Weighted average, 140

ABOUT THE AUTHORS

Stephen Strasser, Ph.D., received his B.A. from the University of Pennsylvania in 1972, and his doctorate from the University of Michigan in 1979. From 1979 to 1981 he taught at Tulane University in both the School of Public Health and Tropical Medicine, and the Business School.

Currently, he is an associate professor in the Division of Hospital and Health Services Administration within the College of Medicine at the Ohio State University. He also holds a joint appointment in the College of Business Administration. Since 1988, he has served as the director of Ohio State's Patient Satisfaction Measurement System Project (PSMS).

Dr. Strasser has authored and coauthored three other books: *Working It Out: Sanity and Success in the Workplace* (Prentice-Hall, 1989), *From Campus to Corporation: And the Next Ten Years* (Career Press, 1990), and *Transitions: Successful Strategies from Mid-Career to Retirement* (Career Press, 1990). He is currently working on a book, titled *Work Is Not a Four-Letter Word* (Business One/Irwin, 1991). Between 1982 and 1988, he wrote a nationally syndicated newspaper column for King Features on human resources management issues that was read by as many as 5 million readers.

Dr. Strasser has published extensively in practitioner and academic journals. His areas of research include the impact of personal control on job satisfaction and job performance, and turnover among health care professionals.

Currently, Dr. Strasser, along with Carson F. Dye, conducts ongoing national seminars for the American College of Healthcare Executives in human resources management. Along with Dr. John Sena, he conducts ongoing College workshops on increasing managerial creativity in health care organizations. He has made over 150 presentations on human resources issues to health care audiences throughout the United States.

Rose Marie "Pinky" Davis received her bachelor's degree from Washington University, St. Louis, in 1970. Her graduate work at the Ohio State University culminated in an M.A. in Asian Art History in 1975. In addition, she completed the Executive Program in Health Care Financial Management at the Ohio State University in 1987. She currently holds an adjunct faculty appointment with the Graduate Program in Hospital and Health Services Administration at the Ohio State University.

While taking Intensive Chinese as a graduate student, she worked part-time as a technician in the cardiology laboratories at the Ohio State University Hospitals. After teaching Asian Art History at Denison University for several years, she pursued a full-time career in health care. For 13 years, she was the administrative director of cardiology at University Hospitals, involved in clinical, research, and teaching programs.

In 1987 a patient relations program was created at the Ohio State University Hospitals. Ms. Davis was hired by the Division of Marketing and Planning as the program's director to define and establish patient relations in this large academic medical center. Recognizing that the cornerstone for a well-integrated program would be knowing clearly what the patients were saying, she formed a collaborative relationship with Stephen Strasser to develop and implement a patient satisfaction measurement system at University Hospitals. This book is the product of their efforts to date.

Ms. Davis is an active member of the National Society of Patient Representation and Consumer Affairs of the American Hospital Association. She has served on national committees and conducted the University Specialty sessions during national meetings. She is also an active member of the Ohio Society for Patient Representatives of the Ohio Hospital Association and has served as a state board member since 1989. She is also a member of the American Academy of Medical Administrators and a nominee for the American College of Healthcare Executives.

In 1990 she developed the curriculum and taught the first three-hour credit course on patient relations to undergraduates in the School of Allied Medical Professions, the Ohio State University.